Ketogenic

MW01489637

Combine the Keto Diet & Nobel Prize Winning Science to Look and Feel Younger, Lose Weight and Extend Your Life + 28 Day OMAD Meal Plan

Written By

Thomas Hawthorn

Thomas Hawthorn

The following eBook is reproduced below with the goal of providing information that is as accurate and reliable as possible. Regardless, purchasing this eBook can be seen as consent to the fact that both the publisher and the author of this book are in no way experts on the topics discussed within and that any recommendations or suggestions that are made herein are for entertainment purposes only. Professionals should be consulted as needed prior to undertaking any of the action endorsed herein.

This declaration is deemed fair and valid by both the American Bar Association and the Committee of Publishers Association and is legally binding throughout the United States.

Furthermore, the transmission, duplication or reproduction of any of the following work including specific information will be considered an illegal act irrespective of if it is done electronically or in print. This extends to creating a secondary or tertiary copy of the work or a recorded copy and is only allowed with an expressed written consent from the Publisher. All additional right reserved.

The information in the following pages is broadly considered to be a truthful and accurate account of facts and as such any inattention, use or misuse of the information in question by the reader will render any resulting actions solely under their purview. There are no scenarios in which the publisher or the original author of this work can be in any fashion deemed liable for any hardship or damages that may befall them after undertaking information described herein.

Additionally, the information in the following pages is intended only for informational purposes and should thus be thought of as universal. As befitting its nature, it is presented without assurance regarding its prolonged validity or interim quality. Trademarks that are mentioned are done without written consent and can in no way be considered an endorsement from the trademark holder.

Medical Disclaimer

This book is not intended as a substitute for the medical advice of physicians. The reader should regularly consult a physician in matters relating to his/her health and particularly with respect to any symptoms that may require diagnosis or medical attention.

Please consult your physician before starting any diet or exercise program.

Any recommendations given in this book are not a substitute for medical advice.

Contents

Introduction

Think of the most popular pairs in history.

Carrot and peas. Salt and pepper. Captain America and Iron Man (or Thor and Hulk for you Asgardian fans). Tom and Hardy. Charlize and Theron.

They go so well together.

And that is exactly what happens when you put autophagy with ketogenesis, they go well together. They complement each other. I do not mean that in a metaphysical or philosophical way. There is a scientific foundation for my conclusions about autophagy and ketogenesis.

But what do the aforementioned terms even mean? I am guessing that to some of you, I might as well have introduced them in Japanese because they are not going to make sense without an explanation.

Well, we are going to explore both autophagy and ketogenesis in depth in a later chapter. For now, what you need to understand is that autophagy helps with the consumption of damaged and dangerous cells. In numerous cases, these cells have the potential to turn cancerous. On the other hand, ketogenesis is the process of creating ketone bodies. These help in distributing energy throughout the body.

How are they related?

Thomas Hawthorn

In a recent study conducted by Japanese scientists on mice, they discovered that when they removed the gene that causes autophagy from the rodents, their ketone levels dropped as well.

Author, you say.

Those are mice, you say. How can they be of significance to us?

There is a reason why laboratories utilize mice in medical testing; they share genetic and biological traits that are close to human beings. It is for this reason that many medicines are first tested out on mice before moving on to human trials.

So far, we do not have any studies about autophagy with ketogenesis performed on humans. Nevertheless, there is an interesting conclusion that one can draw here that intermittent fasting helps with autophagy, which in turn contributes to ketogenesis in the body.

Now you are wondering about the fact that we haven't yet established the connection between fasting and autophagy.

We don't have to.

The US National Library of Medicine National Institutes of Health has done the legwork for us.

According to the world's largest medical library, the ritual of having three meals a day (with a little snacking added in by some people) is not a natural habit and does not provide the human body any benefits. This is because our ancestors – the hunters and the gatherers – did not have the luxury of eating so frequently during the day.

Which is why their bodies would go through a fasting period several times during the day. The body, under the stress of fasting, would, of course, try to protect itself. It did this by removing any cells that could potentially cause the body harm due to the lack of food. This eventually led to the destruction of numerous dangerous cells throughout the body. In short, our ancestors – without having realized it – forced their bodies to cleanse themselves.

In today's world, we are fixated on getting our daily fix of food. This is probably because of the fact that we were taught to have breakfast, lunch, and dinner to stave off hunger. And the practice worked! After all, who likes to stay hungry?

As we grew up, we never really questioned the whole idea of eating so regularly during the day. It never occurred to us that there is a way to have a proper diet that could benefit us and our bodies.

After all, our parents and practically society itself had convinced us to adopt a habit that we never questioned. That is not a bad thing at all. They were concerned about our health and they might not have been aware of autophagy.

However, science has made significant progress during the years. And we can easily become aware of numerous ideas, facts, and studies regarding our health, body, and well-being at the click of a button and a few keystrokes.

Take for example the 2016 Nobel Prize-winning study conducted by Yoshinori Ohsumi, a Japanese cell biologist. He discovered that during fasting, the cells break down various proteins and other materials in our body and turn them into energy. Furthermore, the cells also eliminate invading bacteria and viruses and send them off for recycling. This process of the cell turning materials into energy and recycling harmful components in our body is known as autophagy.

Not many people know about this process, even though it is renowned in the medical community (it won the Nobel Prize after all).

However, if people were made aware of autophagy, then we would have many who would understand just how important intermittent fasting is.

Additionally, when you combine fasting with the ketogenic diet, you are giving the body not only the chance to remove harmful materials but to intake the right materials as well.

See what I mean about how the two processes of autophagy and ketogenesis are an incredible pair?

That is what we shall be focusing on in this book.

I am not here to take you down a confusing labyrinth of complex medical terms and studies. I am here to show you just how important intermittent fasting is for a wholesome life. I am here to give you tips on how you can adopt this method of fasting into your life, how you do not have to give up on your workout regime or fitness routines for the purpose of fasting, and how you can change your life for the better.

I will also guide you through the OMAD, or One Meal a Day, process. You will even learn about why traditional dieting techniques are not exactly benefiting you in any way.

You will become aware of a powerful tool to enable you to unlock the healing potential of your body.

You hold in your hands a compendium that will change the way you see dieting and personal well-being.

On that note, I bid you welcome to the world of Ketogenic Autophagy.

Think of the process as a keto diet on steroids, but instead of causing harm, it is going to cleanse your body.

Chapter 1: Why the Traditional North American Diet is Killing You

You know that when a study involving the eating habits of an entire country becomes newsworthy, then you should probably take notice. Especially if you are residing within said country.

The study we are talking about was conducted by the Journal of the American Medical Association. It garnered so much attention that Time, CBS News, Yahoo!, and even U.S. News covered the topic.

To give to a bit of background and show you the level of seriousness of the study, you need to understand that the results took deep insights from earlier research conducted by the U.S. government for a national health survey. It was no surprise that the survey revealed that most people did not consume the recommended amounts of healthy food.

This led to the Journal of the American Medical Association discovering that what is killing most Americans are their bad eating habits. In fact, the study showed that Americans eat too much bacon, consume too much sugar, and eat too few nuts, vegetables, and fruits. This habit of consuming fatty and sugary foods is truly harmful, leading to heart conditions, diabetes, and even weight gain.

That's right, even sugar can cause weight gain.

How, you ask?

Let us start with why food is important.

Your body depends on food for energy.

We all know that.

But apart from that, the body takes proteins from foods to help the cells in your body do their job. Your body requires the fats from foods to produce new cells and hormones, and help with the movement of vitamins. You are going to need the vitamins from foods if you intend to keep your skin healthy and your bones strong.

In many ways, foods affect many different processes in your body. You need water not just because it makes up to anywhere from 50% to up to 66% of your body weight, but because your body uses it to regulate temperature.

In the same way, foods also affect your weight in more ways than you can imagine.

Take the hormone insulin for example. This hormone is responsible for allowing glucose to enter your cells. Whether you have a healthy dose of insulin or you are taking insulin treatment to regulate the levels of the hormone, the result is the same, insulin sends glucose to your cells and this lowers the amount of glucose in your blood.

The calories that you consume provide the glucose that you require and this is where excess sugar becomes a problem.

If you consume more calories or sugar than required, insulin does not transfer the glucose to your cells. They are simply converted to fats.

The result? Weight gain.

People who suffer from diabetes are at the highest risk of this process. Which is why their doctor or dietician recommends them to provide their body with the right nutrients and minimize the amount of sugar they consume.

But that does not mean non-diabetic people cannot suffer the consequences of a poor diet. In fact, they most probably will.

When we think of a rich or healthy diet, we think of adapting something to fit the typical three-meals-a-day scheme. We are so used to the scheme that we cannot imagine parting with it. In fact, we may have all heard the popular quote "breakfast is the most important meal of the day."

It does sound like it makes sense. In fact, it should be right. Right?

Hardly.

Let me start off by saying that the Romans had it correct.

And no, I am not talking about their politics or economics. I am talking about their meal plan.

Indeed. The Romans had a healthy meal plan, though I am not certain if they had a concept of meal plans back in the day. Let us just say that they had proper eating habits.

Confused? Don't be. It will all make sense in a bit.

First, a bit of background before we revert to the Romans.

The idea of breakfast began with cereal. Before the invention of cereal, people did not consume breakfast as frequently and did not make it part of their routine as they do in the present time.

In fact, during the medieval period, only royalties and people of wealth could enjoy breakfast. It was a luxury back then. Common people could not afford to have meals multiple times during the day. Even having two meals was a treat to those who could not afford them (which practically meant a lot of people).

As time moved on, cities began to develop more and more. Technology brought in convenience and an industrial revolution. Life became much busier. Those employees, workers, and professionals who worked according to a schedule did not receive time to have a decent meal during the day.

Their solution? Might as well have something before heading

off to work. That way, they would not be too hungry.

And lo and behold, we have breakfast getting more common.

Soon, the concept of breakfast spread to different sections of society. This, in turn, gave rise to a whole new market dedicated to serving a new lifestyle of people having meals in the morning.

Eventually, manufacturers realized that people choose foods that they could quickly eat in the morning without having to cook it. Their answer to that? Cereals.

Fun fact: John Harvey Kellogg was one of the people who spearheaded the cereals movement. However, Kellogg's motivations were a bit, unorthodox, to say the least. You see, he believed that cereals could improve the health of people and stop them from desiring masturbation and sex too much. Thankfully, none of his beliefs made it into the marketing campaign or we would be looking at cereals in a completely different light.

So back to cereals.

No, I am not going to say that they actually do play a role in stopping you from enjoying your, well, "me time".

What I will say is that manufacturers needed a hook to sell the cereals. They needed a strong marketing campaign. They focused on convincing people that breakfast is an essential component of your everyday life. They knew that rather than trying to market the product, they could market the idea itself.

It worked. Eventually, this campaign led to numerous messages on the importance of breakfast. You could see stores handing out pamphlets and radio stations proclaiming, "Nutrition experts believe that breakfast is the most essential meal of the day."

The reality, however, is that scientists haven't been able to land on a conclusive answer. Yes, breakfast does help stave off starvation as in many cases, people have not eaten for quite a while (the time difference between lunch and dinner is marginal). However, the idea that breakfast carries most of the burden of keeping you healthy is not the right one.

The breakfast trend created a whole new market that manufacturers took advantage of. In similar ways, the food industry is always keeping an eye out for lifestyle choices and trends that they can use to generate profit.

Over the decades, new food fads keep on rising. As they accumulate, they lead to what we have today: a complex system of food trends where nobody questions the veracity of the facts that they are being bombarded with. Unlike other countries that have relied on agriculture for generations, Americans do not have the support of earlier generations who have lived on growing food for years. This leads to the development of certain ideas about food that may not be grounded on scientific evidence. In fact, new food fads are cropping up even more in the present and people are confused – and in many cases – misled by the information they receive.

New fads arise because they are based on the complex food habits of Americans. These habits are themselves based on the type of foods commonly consumed by the general masses.

And at the base of the food chain (no pun intended) is corn.

Think that is hard to believe?

Let us take some examples of popular foods consumed by Americans.

Gatorade. Hamburgers. Cheetos.

All of these foods are made using compounds created by corn.

In fact, let us take each of the foods listed above and examine how corn influences them.

Gatorade uses corn syrup. Guess what the major content of that ingredient is.

The American cattle industry uses corn heavily. This is because when animals are fed corn, they take less time to fatten. They are, in turn, used as ingredients for some of the most popular foods out there. Chicken patties. Hamburgers.

In fact, think of all the fast food giants like McDonald's, KFC, and Arby's. They need to churn out their products as fast as possible because of the growing demand for their food. To deliver the right amount of supply, they need ingredients such as meat as quickly as possible. This, in turn, encourages industries to use methods to increase the production of meat.

At this point, I don't have to tell you what one of those methods is.

That's right, corn feeding.

What about Cheetos, you ask? Well, some of your favorite snacks are made using enriched corn meal including, you guessed it, Cheetos.

The above three examples that I have provided are just some of the various foods that use corn or a compound of corn.

You might just be thinking, is that all there is to it author? Is that why you are particular about corn?

Far from the truth. In fact, here are a few things you should know about corn in America.

According to SmartMoney, you can find corn in 3 out of every 4 products in the supermarket. Surprised? There is more.

According to data compiled by the U.S. Department of Agriculture, corn is also used by biotech companies. At this point, if you are thinking that perhaps they only consume a little, then think again because the products that use corn as the main input were worth over $125 billion in 2012. Just to give you a sense of scale, the GDP of the country of Angola is predicted by the International Monetary Fund to be around $110 billion in 2019. Think about it, the biotech industry is just one of the many industries that utilize corn. Imagine if we start to combine every industry dependent on corn. This goes to show just how much industries depend on the cereal grain.

According to the National Corn Growers Association, Americans consume more than one-third of all the corn produced in the world. This fact can be combined with another study which has shown that many Americans can attribute over 50 percent of their biomass to corn!

Why am I stating these facts? For one, when so many people depend on corn to such a high degree, then there are definitely going to be brands, companies, and manufacturers ready to meet their demands through various corn-based products. For another, no matter how many facts we present to the world, we might find ourselves facing the growing number of products on the supermarket shelf to show that we might not be getting anywhere with our fact-checks. In fact, when industries realize that science might hamper their profit line, they hire lobbyists to ensure that their production is not threatened. They create a type of "carb craze" to keep people going after their products time and time again. You might not even be aware that this phenomenon of "carb craze" is taking place. When you only see the end results – which are the numerous products available in the market – that are available in your local store or supermarket, it can be difficult to imagine that most of those products are fueled by corn. But that alone is what fuels Americans' dependency on these high carb content products.

Of course, no one would ever manufacture their products under the title of "high" carbs".

I am not sure if people would run after their products if they did something like that.

Nowadays, manufacturers have another food fad or trend that they are after. In fact, you might have seen many products with a special label – low carbs.

That label makes everything sound healthy. People who are looking to reduce their carb consumption are probably thinking what a great alternative low-carb foods can make.

However, those labels are just what they are and nothing more; they are merely labels. You see, if you buy a product that has the label "low carb", there is no assurance that it has a much lower carbohydrate content than other products or foods that do not have such a label. Why is that? Because there are no nutrition cataloging guidelines or legal classifications for low-carbohydrate foods. This means that is it entirely up to the manufacturer to decide what exactly they think low-carb means. And the best part? Low-carb foods are more expensive!

Here is an example: when you purchase a low-carb beer, you are going to consume about 2.6 grams of carbohydrates. When you perform a rough calculation, the whole content of the beer equals 95 calories. If you choose a regular light beer, you are going to consume about 3.2 grams of carbohydrates. That amounts to about 96 calories. For such a dismal amount of difference, you are paying almost 50% to 75% more than your average light beer.

When a new food trend appears, you have an entire industry pouncing upon it to make the most use of it. They want you to purchase their products. They definitely do not want you to adopt a keto diet. Why would they? If you practiced eating healthy food and combine it with intermittent fasting, then who is going to consume all the variety of carb-filled (or so-called "low carb") foods stacked one above the other on your local supermarket shelf?

Over the years, manufacturers have adopted various techniques to sell their products and defend their stance against the growing concern about the ingredients they utilize. Apart from the aforementioned low-carb labels that they attach to their products, they have also gone on to spread information about the harmful effects of proteins. The popular theory is that proteins cause the load of acid in your body to increase. This, in turn, compels the body to take in calcium from your bones to neutralize the acidity levels. The increase in calcium causes problems in your kidneys, a notable example is the formation of kidney stones.

In reality, long-term studies have disproved this idea.

These studies have found that protein intake does not harm the bones and definitely does not damage the kidneys. The opposite is true. Proteins have been known to improve bone density! Let us also not forget the fact that proteins are the building blocks of life! How else do you imagine your cells functioning if they do not have the support of proteins?

You have the power to make informed decisions about your life. You have to understand what information is true and what is just manufactured to make sure you do not change your bad habits.

We just saw how bad habits are affecting the health of an entire nation. We also saw how habits are formed and how manufacturers make use of those habits (also called food fads or trends in the modern jargon) to sell you items that you probably do not need in your life.

Which is why we have a keto diet as your savior.

Chapter 2: Ketosis Without the BS

Let's get the obvious out of the way:

A keto diet is a low-carb and high-fat diet.

You use this diet to make sure that your body burns fat more effectively.

More than 50 studies have been conducted on the diet and results show that the diet benefits a plethora of areas: weight loss, better health, improved physical performance, and more.

Now that is out of the way, let us look at some of the things you might not be aware of about a keto diet. More importantly, what exactly is happening to your body on a daily basis? Sure, you are getting healthier, but shouldn't there be more details?

There are.

When you are on a keto diet, you tend to feel less hungry. Eventually, your body starts producing ketones. Ketones, in turn, assist your body in controlling hormones that affect your appetite. They control the influence of hormones like ghrelin, which is your "hunger" hormone. While doing so, they also enhance the production of cholecystokinin, which is the hormone that gives you the feeling of being "full" or less hungry.

When you combine keto diet's effects on the above hormones, you have a wonderful result. You do not feel like snacking regularly. When we are hungry, we tend to consume whatever we get our hands on. In our minds, we feel that we are merely snacking a small amount to manage our hunger. However, when you add up the little snacks you have been consuming over a period of time such as a month, then you might just notice an alarming result: you have consumed a whopping amount of snacks in total!

A keto diet controls your habit of grabbing small bites regularly, making it easier for you to go longer without food.

Your body then has to reach out to other sources for its energy. Enter your fat reserves. When your body starts consuming your fat, you start losing weight fairly quickly.

But hold on just a minute. Didn't we just say that we are going to focus on a high-fat diet in keto? So are we losing weight just to gain it back?

That is not true.

First of all, let us get something out of the way. Fats are not bad. Your body needs fats. The problem occurs when you consume too much of them.

In a keto diet, you are consuming the right amount of good fats at a specific time in the day, avoiding three-meal a day schemes and unnecessary snacking.

You consume plenty of good fats on a keto diet. This fat helps you remain satiated, preventing you from feeling hunger quickly. Fat also stabilizes your blood sugar levels and prevents you from experiencing extreme fluctuations in your energy levels.

When your body functions by using ketones as a source of fuel, then it has a stable energy source. On the other hand, when your body uses carbs it requires frequent doses of carbs to keep it functioning normally.

Think of the times that you eat a big pack of chips to stave of hunger. You might have eaten the entire pack by yourself but you still find yourself hungry a couple of hours later. Sometimes even sooner. When some people experience this form of hunger, they brush it off thinking that they probably consumed a small number of chips. Far from it. It is not the number of chips that caused the hunger. It is the body's growing dependence on carbs.

When you transition from these carb-filled foods to a keto diet with useful fats, you can power through the day without feeling the need to stare at your refrigerator the way a hungry hyena stares at its new prey.

But to reap the benefits of a keto diet, you cannot expect changes to occur overnight. There is a process that takes place.

Keto-adaption is a multifaceted process. Your body is shifting from the use of glucose, as it has been doing for years, to primarily utilizing ketones and the fat it stores for energy. Your body needs time to accommodate that change. Your body might require longer than a few days to get used to the process.

If you look at the changes occurring on a day-to-day basis, then here is what happens. After two to four days, the blood ketone levels in your body might increase to anywhere from 1 to 2 millimolar, or mM. A millimolar is a measurement used to show how concentrated something is in a solution. During this phase, it might be rather difficult for people to maintain keto's low-carb diet.

Sometimes, it might be more challenging for certain people to adapt to a keto diet. In such cases, they might have to reduce their carb intake even further.

At this point, you might wonder if you can simply make use of any low carb diet. Does that not equate to entering into a state of ketosis?

The reality is far more complex than that.

First, let us seek to understand the difference between a keto diet and a low-carb diet by examining each one independently.

Understanding the Keto Diet

In a ketogenic diet, you are pushing your body to use as few carbs as it can. In many ways, people split their diet into a ratio that shows the percentage of fat, protein, and carbs they consume in a particular day. Generally, the division of nutrients happens in the below percentage:

- Fat: 65% to 80%

- Protein: 15% to 25%

- Carbs: 5% to 10%

Yikes. You might not have been expecting your carb levels to drop that low. But welcome to the keto diet and quite frankly, every part of the diet is necessary. And no, there is no wiggle room for change. You are not going to get an 11% carb rate or a 12% carb rate. However, do note that the ratio of carbohydrates may vary depending on the situation or the diet.

For most people, adopting a keto diet means having below 50 grams of carbs per day. By drastically reducing your intake of carbs, you coax your body into a state of ketosis which then becomes the process that provides the main source of fuel for your body.

Essentially, the percentage split in the diet that I had mentioned earlier meant that:

- You are going to have mostly fat until you are satisfied.

- You are going to get your protein intake because it is essential (do not pay heed to the rumor mill about its harmful effects).

- You are also going to get a small number of calories from carbohydrates.

Through the process of ketosis, you are entering into a unique metabolic state that acts as a response to an energy crisis. The only difference is that you are going to respond to that crisis by ensuring that you have the right materials to supply. Basically, you are changing the selection of fuel for your body. You are taking away something that is not good for you and adding something that benefits you greatly.

Understanding the Low-Carb Diet

One of the primary differences that you can make out between a keto diet and a low-carb diet is that in a low-carb diet, there are no strict levels of carbs you should consume in a day. The idea is to reduce the intake of carbs but there is no specific limit.

Low-carb diets are typically not so low that they push your body in a state of full ketosis. You might enter a mild form of ketosis between your low-carb meals. But remember, that state of mild ketosis only lasts until your next meal. You are going to exit the state real quick. For the most part, you won't enter a full-ketosis mode on a low-carb diet. However, there are certain exceptions to this rule. When you are sleeping, perform a fast, or workout, to highlight a few examples, you might enter into a more intense state of ketosis. However, do note that you more than likely won't be taking advantage of the ketosis process through a low-carb diet. This is because when you enter a specific state and exit it quickly you are not taking advantage of the process. You have to enter ketosis and make sure that you maintain that state for a long period of time and as frequently as possible.

That does not mean that there are no easy techniques or steps you can take to achieve full ketosis. Here are the main tips that you need to be aware of to enter into a state of ketosis:

- The most important part is to minimize your carb intake as much as possible. Remember the 5% to 10% split? That should be your starting point. You could start off at 10% carbs and then reduce as you see fit.

- Try to include coconut oil in your diet. This is because it contains certain fats called medium-chain triglycerides (MCTs). What is different about this fat? Well, MCTs can be easily used by the liver. Once they enter the liver, they can be used as a source of energy or can be turned to ketones. Here is an interesting fact about coconut oil. Research has also shown that consuming coconut oil can be one of the best methods to increase the level of ketones for Alzheimer's disease patients. People with nervous system disorders can also make use of coconut oil to improve ketone levels.

- Increase your physical activity. There are two main reasons for this. One is that ketosis helps you perform better in numerous physical activities, including endurance based sports. The other reason is that physical activities, in turn, help you enter ketosis. It is a wonderful balance and helps you make the most of your diet.

- I mentioned good fats before. You should be focusing on taking in more of such fats. You will need them as a source of energy after all.

- Maintain a proper level of protein intake. Do not consume too much of it. Now, you might think to yourself that what the big companies have been saying was true all along, protein is not good for you. That is not the reason I asked you to maintain your protein intake. Too much of anything is bad for you. Too many carbs? Bad for you. Too much sugar? Definitely not recommended. Too much calcium? You are going to feel the effects of that. In a similar manner, you need to control your protein intake as well. However, the fact still remains that protein is vital for your body.

With all of this mention of keto and low-carb diets, you may wonder how you are going to know if you are actually in a state of ketosis or if you are simply in the process of being on just another diet.

Is there a test to determine the level of ketosis?

As a matter of fact, there is.

If you have heard of the procedure where people utilize strips to take a ketosis test, let me tell you that you won't have to do the same.

Here are a few tell-tale signs:

Breath

When you begin your keto journey, you might experience what people commonly call "keto breath". When your body begins to produce ketone bodies, one of the byproducts of the process is acetone. The smell of this byproduct is rather unique. Some people claim to smell "nail polish" while others claim it has a distinct "fruity" or "metallic" smell to it.

Whatever scent you get from acetone, it stays for just the first few weeks and then disappears after that. You can minimize its effect by brushing or flossing, but you probably won't be able to remove the smell completely.

Weight Loss

Your weight loss might not come as a surprise to you. After all, losing any extra weight is something that we would like to achieve as well. You can experience a fast drop in weight within the first week itself. Many people falsely believe that this happens due to the loss of fat, the reality is that it is the result of the body using up the stored carbs and water.

After the initial drop in your weight, you should notice a continual decrease in your body fat as long as you maintain a state of deficiency in your calorie intake.

Decreased Hunger

Once you are well into a ketogenic diet, you might experience a reduction in your hunger levels. This is a good reaction to the diet. When you do not feel hungry too often, you are not compelled to start thinking about getting a small snack. Though the research behind your decreased hunger is sparse, scientists are still trying to figure out just what causes a keto diet to help you prevent feeling the urge to nibble on some goodies frequently.

Increased Energy

When people adopt a low-carb diet (and not a keto diet), they often report feeling tired and sick easily. However, people who take up a keto diet have noticed increased levels of focus and energy. Do note that it does take a while for you to get

Thomas Hawthorn

used to the diet and notice its effects.

Short-Term Fatigue

When you switch to a keto diet, the initial phase (which comprises the first few weeks), might be the most challenging for people. One of the effects that many people feel is fatigue and weakness.

People who go through such effects often feel like they would prefer quitting the diet altogether. In many cases, people do indeed give up on the diet.

But here is something you should know about the keto diet: fatigue in the beginning is completely normal. Your body has spent decades getting used to one particular diet filled with carbohydrates and now it has to make a switch to another diet devoid of the regular supply of carbs. It is similar to writing using one hand for half your life and then trying to write with the other hand, hoping to master the process in just a single day. It is not going to happen. You need time to get over the initial discomfort before you can make any progress.

The same train of thought applies to a keto diet as well. You might feel discomfort initially, but do not give up on your new food habits. Go along with it for a few weeks and allow your body to acclimatize itself to the new shift in your eating habits.

After all, the end result is worth the change.

Chapter 3: The Relationship Between Ketosis and Autophagy

Did you know that in Greek, the word autophagy actually means to eat one's self?

That sounds rather barbaric, doesn't it? One might think that anything associated with that word is dastardly.

However, there is some truth to the Greek meaning of the word when you use it to describe the process occurring within the body.

When there are no external supplies of food, the body begins to eat itself. However, it does not do this in a horrific way. What actually happens is that your body targets damaged proteins and cells. By destroying these components, the process gives way for newer and healthier cells and proteins to arise in their place.

You are encouraging your body to regenerate.

Doesn't the body always get rid of damaged cells?

It does.

But as we age, we experience stress, more physical activities, burnouts, and other constant pressures of everyday life. This increases the rate at which the cells in our bodies begin to deteriorate. Add the fact that we are feeding our body unhealthy components, and we are not giving it enough of a break to take care of the damaged cells.

This is why autophagy is important: It helps to remove the increasing number of damaged cells from the body, including certain types of cells called senescent cells that have no actual purpose other than lingering inside organs and tissues. One of the main reasons to ensure that we remove damaged and senescent cells from our body is because these cells can activate inflammatory pathways and could become vital factors in the formation of various diseases.

We are better off without them.

Autophagy is not just a weapon against bad cells. You can use it to obtain a lot of advantages for your body. Here are just a few of them.

Bodily Function and Quality of Life

You might have heard the term "anti-aging" being thrown around a lot. It does have its charms and many products claim to provide you with the ability to turn back the clock on your body. Well, that is not entirely possible. However, autophagy has a way to make a type of anti-aging process occur within your body. How does it happen? Since the early 1950s, scientists have been aware of the process of autophagy but it was only recently that they were able to uncover more information about how it improves the health of your cells by replacing the damaged ones, as we had seen before. This process results in the following:

Newer cells mean healthier cells. This means your bodily functions improve tremendously.

When your cells are repaired or replaced, they function much better. This, in turn, means that they behave like newer and younger cells. When they do, you feel and look younger.

Increased Longevity

The above point directly links to another benefit that autophagy provides the body: longevity. When you are replacing damaged cells with healthier (and younger) ones, then you are preventing older cells from taking over your body. When you have old cells, they not only function slowly but they also cause your body to slack and age slightly faster. Think of the times you have seen many people say that they are in their 40s or 50s and you are taken aback simply because they do not look their age. The reason for their youthful appearance and vigor is no miracle product or treatment. It is simply the body getting rid of older proteins and cells. Is autophagy similar to the fountain of youth? Nothing so dramatic I'm afraid. But autophagy does come pretty close to making you feel and look young, minus any invasive procedures.

Reducing Chronic Inflammation

Autophagy helps your body manage its level of inflammation by either boosting or suppressing the degree of immune response that you might require for a given situation. For the most part, autophagy reduces the inflammation caused by your immune response by managing the proteins called antigens that give the signals that activate such responses.

Preventing and Delaying Neurodegenerative Diseases

According to the US National Library of Medicine National Institutes of Health, many neurodegenerative diseases are caused by damaged, or what scientists call "misfolded", proteins. As we have seen how autophagy gets rid of these damaged proteins, the process eventually reduces the severity of various neurodegenerative diseases such as Alzheimer's disease. In many cases, autophagy has also been known to prevent the spread of such diseases across the brain.

Autophagy is our body's superpower. It is the way we can improve our vitality while staving off diseases and health complications. But where does ketosis fit into all of this? How does intermittent fasting lead to better autophagy? Why have celebrities such as Beyonce and Hugh Jackman all gone public about the benefits of keto dieting?

Let us take it from the top once again.

We have already established how fasting helps your body

enter a state of ketosis. This way, you are avoiding the dependency on carbs and instead relying on the useful fats that you consume during the fasting period. The process of using useful fat helps your body release chemicals called ketones. The ketones have an important role to play in your brain, where they release an essential protein called Brain-derived neurotrophic factor, or BDNF. One of the many purposes of BDNF is to build and reinforce neurons and neural pathways in those areas of the brain that are focused on memory and learning. This is probably why a lot of people claim to have a better capacity to retain information and an improved learning process when they enter a keto diet.

So far, so good. We have fasting based on a keto diet releasing all the good stuff in your body.

We have also seen how fasting triggers autophagy and gets rid of the harmful proteins and cells in your body. But when you add ketosis to the equation, then what really happens is that you remove your body's dependency on carbs. You see, carbs actually delay the autophagy process by days because they are your body's primary source of fuel. They cannot be recycled quickly enough.

Ketosis, on the other hand, increases the use of fats. This, in turn, makes the body less dependent on carbs. Which means you do not feel compelled to eat as often as you used to. And when you can manage your eating habits, your body is ready to enter the autophagy phase. You are then ready to eat less and live better.

And that is how the magic happens.

Nevertheless, we often look at calories like a criminal that needs to be given a life sentence. They are not completely bad. In fact, if you are aiming to lose weight, then you have to make note of something important: calories are units of energy. When you take the factor of energy into consideration, then you should realize your body does need energy. It just needs a calorie deficit diet to provide with enough energy to keep you going while you use up the energy in your fat stores. You are avoiding excess and adopting the rule of moderation. You still need calories to help you with processes such as maintaining your body heat.

In fact, you cannot completely remove energy from your body. If you do that, then you are violating the first rule of thermodynamics, which simply states that the internal work that is performed by the system has to equal the work that is done by that system. This means that you need just enough calories to ensure that you do not disrupt your body's normal functions or work.

Ketosis and autophagy cannot simply override or replace that.

Chapter 4: Surprising Benefits of One Meal a Day (OMAD)

When you have a culture saturated with the idea of excess, especially when it comes to food, then you have people trying to look for alternatives. When people become aware of the harmful effects of consuming too much of something, they realize that they should look for a method that might help them not just curb their habits, but bring their body into a better state.

At this point, people look to various dieting and fasting routines including your friendly neighborhood intermittent fasting.

At its core, intermittent fasting is beneficial to your body. You lose weight. You increase the rate at which fats are burned. You lower the levels of insulin and sugar in your bloodstream. You could even reverse the effects of type 2 diabetes.

With all of these advantages, intermittent fasting sounds like the ideal technique to focus on. While that may be true, intermittent fasting may not provide all the benefits that you might be seeking from the process. In other words, it is simply just not enough. Intermittent fasting has some incredible benefits when you look at the short-term, but it cannot guarantee benefits over a long period of time. And here is why.

In intermittent fasting, you are going without food anywhere from 12 to 16 hours. At the end of the period, you are going to eat food that benefits you. You are going to fill yourself with the right nutrients and the right amount of fats. You are ideally looking to lose as much weight as possible, remove harmful cells from your body, and live a long life with as many physical and mental benefits as you can possibly attain.

With intermittent fasting, you are not giving your body enough time to completely enter ketosis and bring about the process of autophagy. This is because, by the time the processes kick in, you have already provided food and nourishment to your body. You delay the processes slightly more.

This does not mean that intermittent fasting is not useful or does not work. It does! But we are looking to get your body into a healthier state of being through a much better method that sustains your health over a long period of time.

And is there such a method for you to use?

There is.

Let me introduce you to OMAD.

In OMAD fasting, you are aiming for a 23:1 ratio or a 20:4 ratio. What does this mean? Well, you are allowing your body between 20 and 23 hours every day to take advantage of the fasting process. You could be using the process for numerous reasons, maybe you aim to burn fat, improve your mental focus and attention, reduce your dependency on harmful foods, or simply help your body remove those compounds that are causing it harm. Whatever your reasons are when you begin to live on one meal a day you are taking your keto diet to the next level.

Fasting techniques such as OMAD boost your body by triggering stress response pathways that enhance the performance of your mitochondria (the organelle in the cell that is responsible for energy production), kick start the autophagy process, and improve the repair of DNA in your cells. OMAD also activates useful metabolic changes and reduces the risk of getting a chronic disease.

Apart from the above benefits, OMAD is known to increase your tolerance to hunger and allows your body to burn more fat for longer periods. OMAD also adds the benefit of lowering your blood sugar levels better than intermittent fasting. It increases the function of the insulin in your body. When you combine lowered blood sugar levels and improved insulin function, then you can reduce obesity much more effectively than any other form of fasting.

When you combine this with your keto diet, you are creating a method that helps you improve on the benefits that intermittent fasting can provide.

You are creating the ultimate form of fasting.

You are ready to be the Jedi knight of fasting.

Of course, there is much to learn before that so let us strap in. We are now going to find out just why OMAD is so good for us.

- For one, you are building a certain type of hormone called Human Growth Hormone, or HGH. This hormone serves plenty of purposes, but the benefit that we are most interested in at this point is the fact that HGH helps in building muscles. This is important to know because many people are of the opinion that OMAD has a negative impact on the development of muscles. According to the US National Library of Medicine National Institutes of Health, it doesn't. Not even close.

- Remember the inflammatory levels that we were talking about? Well, turns out that you can reduce those levels faster through this fasting method.

- And who can forget those nasty diseases? OMAD makes certain that you are reducing the risk of neurodegenerative diseases and it does so much better than intermittent fasting.

- Oh and the best part? OMAD increases the autophagy pathways in our body. What does this mean? You have better autophagy, leading to a better system for eradicating cells and proteins that your body does not require.

If intermittent fasting is the Bruce Banner of fasting, then having a single meal a day is like having the power of the Hulk. You are going to have so much more energy and the fasting itself is going to be so much more powerful and potent.

Then again, what does that mean? How can we translate the power and energy that you feel into benefits that you can see in your lifestyle? What are the changes that you are going to notice in your life that visibly show that your OMAD diet is working?

Here are some of those changes or improvements:

Increased Productivity

The initial shift to one meal a day is not without its challenges. But that is to be expected. You are making a big leap into another territory that gives you numerous benefits but also cuts back on a lot of the calories and carbs that you have been consuming so far. After successfully conquering the first phase of the diet, you are then going to notice changes in your ability. You might find your energy levels increasing. You are going to be more productive during the day.

Laser-Like Focus

Every meal that you are going to consume is going to have the right amount of energy and the right nutrients for your body. You are going to avoid any compounds that are going to have a negative effect on your life. Eventually, as you digest your food, you are going to send all that energy throughout your body, increasing your focus, attention span, and even brain activity. You are going to not just live better, but perform better!

Mental Clarity

If you have worked in an office setting, then you might be aware of your co-workers often talking about having lunch or making breakfast plans. Food is obviously an integral part of our lives. However, in many cases, it becomes a component that seeks to grab our attention at multiple times during the day. We might be engaged in an activity and might suddenly find thoughts of food swirling in our head. We might try and ignore those thoughts but we know that eventually, we are going to cave in to the temptation and order food or cook something for ourselves. OMAD helps you control those urges. You are getting everything you require in one meal so you do not feel the compulsion to grab a bite when you least expect it.

Chapter 5: Exercising Around OMAD

When you are adopting a healthy lifestyle, being active and having a plan to include exercises or workout sessions in your day becomes an essential part of that lifestyle. The scheduling or timing of your exercises can impact the outcome on your one meal a day plan, especially if you find yourself already managing your hunger. There are also many other components to take into consideration depending on the goals and objectives of your exercises or workouts.

Here is something you should make a note of, when your body enters a state of fasting it burns off the sugar it has stored and then moves on to the fat. It breaks down the fat and then converts it into ketones as a source of fuel for the body.

But why does this happen during a fasting state?

It has to do with insulin. When your body has received food or when you have entered a state of feeding, the levels of insulin increases in the body. Insulin is known to regulate the breakdown of fat and numerous research studies have shown that an increase in insulin levels has been shown to control fat metabolism by up to 22%.

During a fasting state, you are controlling the levels of insulin in your body which in turn increases the breakdown of fat.

Additionally, when you work out during fasting, you can start to see an improvement in an area you might not have thought of before, depression. That is right. Combine your workouts with the reduced levels of insulin and you can regulate your mental state much better than before. You are less likely to encounter sudden shifts in your mood or state of mind.

This, in turn, helps you keep your mind active and focused. Your brain spends less time dealing with the effects of depression and stress, which means that you are keeping it healthy.

Let us take a look at a few tips and common concerns about exercises and workouts while adopting an OMAD plan.

What to Consider

- Time your workouts. Do not exercise for periods longer than 60 minutes.

- Keep yourself hydrated. Ensure that you consume water before, during, and after your exercises.

- Your body is one of your best indicators. If you feel weak or nauseated during your workouts, then do not continue further. A recommendation would be to consult with your physician to adjust your food and workout schedules in a way that could benefit you greatly.

- If you are engaged in intense exercises or weight training, then having your one meal of the day after your workouts becomes important. Consider arranging your workout plans accordingly

- Take into consideration factors such as when you last ate, your age, whether or not you are pregnant, your medical history, whether you are taking any medications, your current fitness level, and even your body mass. These factors help you decide the right type of exercise for your OMAD plans.

- Make sure that you are consuming food that is high in protein and contains good fats. Include non-starchy vegetables in your diet. We are going to talk more about the diet that you need to follow during OMAD in the next chapter.

What to Avoid

- Working out for more than 60 minutes.

- Working out if you have a medical condition.

- Performing intense exercises when you have low blood sugar levels.

- Eating meals rich in carbohydrates as it could set the stage for frequent bouts of hunger.

- Working out in the mornings. Morning workouts are a common practice among many people as it allows them to utilize the remaining hours of the day to do other things. Exercising in the mornings can also be a common practice among those people who have certain work schedules or family obligations. However, while in the process of OMAD, you remain in a state of fasting until your eating period arrives later during the day. This can be a challenge mentally because you might end up waiting a long time before you eat.

Let us take an example to illustrate this. You have set your eating schedule anywhere between 3 pm to 7 pm (as people typically schedule their eating periods in the evening). If you work out in the morning at around 9 am, then you will end up waiting for another five to eight hours before you can actually have your meal. That might be rather uncomfortable. Waiting for your eating period to arrive can be challenging enough for you, but throw in your morning exercises and you will only increase your hunger.

So when exactly is the right time to work out during the OMAD process?

The ideal exercising time is just before you have your one meal.

Taking the above example, if you are planning to have your one meal at 5 pm, then you should ideally plan your workouts around 3 or 4 pm. What you are trying to do is keep at least an hour difference between the time you conclude exercising and the time you are about to have your meal.

Of course, some people may not be able to schedule their exercises only in the evenings. What if you only have time in the mornings? Is there a way you can still make use of an OMAD diet?

There is definitely a way. You can use any of the below liquids:

Water

You should especially aim to have mineral water. There is a reason for the word "mineral" to appear in the phrase as numerous minerals are added to the liquid. The percentage of minerals may vary from one mineral water to another, so make sure you read the label to pick out the one you prefer.

One of the unsung heroes in the list of components in mineral water is sulfates.

Sulfur is the eighth most common component of your body in terms of mass. Your body cannot utilize sulfates by directly consuming sulfur. For that reason, you need to consume foods that contain sulfate. Your solution? Mineral water.

Coffee

One of the biggest advantages of having coffee during an

OMAD diet is its ability to control your appetite. Additionally, since you are fasting, the coffee tends to have an even greater effect, supplying your body with even more energy.

Caffeine also releases a neurotransmitter in the brain called dopamine. Dopamine plays a vital role in your emotional and mental well-being. This means that having coffee improves your mood, increases your focus, and improves your productivity.

Bone Broth

This is highly recommended in small doses. Research conducted on obese people has shown that their bodies contain large amounts of a type of bacteria called Firmicutes. The research has also shown that Firmicutes help with extracting high amounts of calories from food. When you drink bone broth, you also consume high amounts of a certain compound known as L-glutamine. One of the most important functions of L-glutamine is to lower the number of Firmicutes in the stomach, eventually aiding in weight loss.

There are people who might complete their workout during the afternoons. If you are one of those people, then worry not. There is a schedule you can follow as well. Instead of keeping your mealtime during the evening, try and adjust it to your workout schedule. For example, if you are going to work out at 1 pm then your one meal of the day should be scheduled anywhere between 2:30 pm to 3 pm, depending on the length of your workout session.

Another question that is asked frequently when it comes to fasting is about the intake of BCAA. People who are engaged in regular workouts are sometimes known to take branched-chain amino acid supplements. So does taking these supplements break your fast?

The short answer is, yes it does.

Essentially, BCAA's are supplements that contain numerous micronutrients. One of the main components of BCAA are amino acids and these amino acids contain fairly high doses of proteins. Which is why, whether you consume BCAAs in tablet or powder form, you are still taking in nutrients that you are supposed to gain from your single meal of the day.

Furthermore, BCAAs also contain calories. This calorie content upsets the balance that you are trying to attain through your OMAD plan. You might still require BCAA depending on the goals you are trying to achieve through your workout routines.

For example, you could be:

- Building muscle

- Performing weight training

- Preparing for a bodybuilding contest

- Training for a physically demanding and competitive sport or feat of endurance

In such cases, you might have to take in BCAA to provide you the type of results you are seeking. If you are simply aiming to lose weight and attain a healthier lifestyle, then you do not have to include BCAA as part of your food intake.

Optimal Cardiovascular Training on OMAD

What exactly is a cardiovascular training or exercise?

Cardiovascular exercise aims to increase your heart and breathing rate to moderate or intense levels for a specific time. Typically, fitness coaches recommend raising the heartbeat for about 10 minutes or more. However, we are not going to aim to keep the heart rate high for longer periods (remember, you are on an OMAD diet). Some of the more common forms of cardio activities people engage in are jogging, running, brisk walking, swimming, cycling, and rowing. If you are headed for the gym, then you might find numerous cardio machines that include the treadmill, gym cycles, stepping machine, and more.

For your cardiovascular training, here are the steps you can follow:

Warm Up and Stretching

Make sure you warm up to get your blood flowing. Warm-ups

are like the lubricants added to vehicles to smoothen the engines, they relax your muscles and allow you to move your body without much resistance.

Begin by carrying out a warmup for roughly five to ten minutes. Keep the warm-up at a low intensity. You are only trying to prep your muscles for the session and gradually increase your heart rate.

Next, start performing activities that raise your heart rate to about 50 to 60% of its maximum rate. You can use any activity to perform your workout. You could even use the treadmill. If you are opting to run or walk, begin by running or walking at a relaxed pace that gets you to this heart rate. You should have a nice, quick heart rate going and still be able to talk about the last season of Game of Thrones with your friend.

Finally, time to stretch. Work on the muscles you will be focusing on in your workout. Warm them up and then utilize stretches to increase their flexibility. If there are special routines for the muscle group you are going to focus on during your workout, then take advantage of those routines.

Frequency of Exercises

As you are dieting, research into fitness has shown that performing cardiovascular exercises for 150 minutes every week is beneficial to your health. You need to take part in moderate-intensity exercises or activities. Make sure that you are spreading out the workout sessions throughout the week instead of clustering them too close together.

Here is a tip from the American College of Sports Medicine. They recommend that you carry out cardiovascular exercises roughly three to five days a week. They further suggest giving your body the time to build and repair the muscles. Therefore, you could carry out the exercises on alternate days.

Duration of Exercises

Finally, we arrive at the most important question: how long is too long? Well, when you are engaged in cardiovascular exercises, you should ideally aim for anywhere between 20 to 60 minutes, based on your capacity and your goals. You should keep your heart rate within the level of intensity that I mentioned earlier. Do not try to work out beyond the 60-minute mark or you might feel faint or dizzy.

The Benefits of Exercising with OMAD

Based on a study conducted by the Healthy Active Living and Obesity Research Group at the University of Ottawa in Canada, overweight people who performed just 150 minutes of low to moderate exercises on a weekly basis lived nearly 4 years longer than overweight people who did not have any exercise routines in their lives.

This study reveals a lot about the importance of exercise. When you combine this benefit of exercise with the longevity you are gaining through OMAD, you have a perfect combination of habits that you need to incorporate in your life. Your one meal diet and your workout routines complement each other wonderfully to give you a fulfilled life.

And the best part is? You do not have to engage in strenuous activities or high-intensity workouts. You just need to walk. In fact, as an alternative to working out at the gym, you could choose to enjoy the outdoors through a brisk walking session.

Men and women are encouraged to add regular exercises into their lives. While it is true that workouts affect men and women differently, the situation only occurs for high-intensity workouts. When you engage in a low to moderate intensity activities or workouts, then you are performing the same activity regardless of your gender.

For example, men can lift much quicker than women. Which is why women may often focus on other forms of exercises.

However, when you are walking briskly, jogging, or using the treadmill, it does not matter whether you arc male or female, you can take advantage of the exercise.

Resistance

You can also take advantage of resistance exercises. When

you perform any exercise to move your body against a source of resistance, then you are involved in strength or resistance training. You can add resistance to your body by moving your body against gravity or by using certain objects to create resistance. Examples of such objects could be dumbbells. Various machines at the gym also add resistance to your body.

Not many people are used to resistance workouts. It might take them a while to adapt to the changes that these workouts can cause to your muscles. If you are new to resistance exercises, then you can make use of certain programs to help you get started.

I recommend the basic program by Alexander Juan Antonio Cortes' Foundations Program to be ideal for your requirements. If you are interested in the workout, head over to his website or type this address into your browser - https://cortes.site/foundations-program/

Calisthenics

Another type of exercise that you can take advantage of during your OMAD diet is calisthenics. Simply put, calisthenics is bodyweight training. When you make any movement that makes use of your body weight and nothing else, then you are performing calisthenics.

Here are a few different types of workouts that you can

incorporate in your daily life for various purposes.

No Equipment Calisthenics

You have to perform four cycles of the below workouts:

- Squats – 8

- Lunges – 8

- Push-ups – 8

- Laying Down Leg Raises – 8

- Plank - If you are a beginner to planks, then simply hold them for 30 seconds. Increase the time as you improve.

- Pike Push-ups – 8

- Mountain Climbers – As many as possible (you can stick to about 20 climbers for each leg when you are starting out).

Basic Beginner Workout

You have to perform four cycles of the below workouts:

- Close Hands Chin Ups – 7

- Pull-ups – 5

- Dips – 6

- Push-ups – 15

- Laying Down Leg Raises – 8

- Jump Squats – 9

Fat Removal Workout

You have to perform four cycles of the below workouts:

- Run – 100 meters

- Dips – 5

- Jumping Jacks – 45 seconds

- Push-ups – 8

- Mountain climbers – 30 seconds

- Planks – 15 seconds

When you are carrying out the above exercises, make sure you schedule them on alternate days. Let us take an example of a schedule. Let us assume that you have chosen to work on the Basic Beginner Workout. Your schedule could look like this:

- Monday: Workout

- Tuesday: Rest Day

- Wednesday: Workout

- Thursday: Rest Day

- Friday: Workout

- Saturday: Workout

- Sunday: Rest Day

You can also combine different exercises to attain various results. For example, you could create a schedule such as the below:

- Monday: Basic Beginner Workout

- Tuesday: No Equipment Calisthenics

- Wednesday: Rest Day

- Thursday: Fat Removal Workout

- Friday: Rest Day

- Saturday: Basic Beginner Workout/Fat Removal Workout/ No Equipment Calisthenics (alternate between the three every week)

- Sunday: Rest Day

You can modify the above routine as you see fit. The idea is to make sure that you are giving your body the exercise it deserves along with your OMAD diet. This helps in creating a complete benefit package for your body.

Make sure that you are comfortable with the workouts. If you feel like you are on the verge of losing consciousness, then do not push yourself to continue further. Remember that you are giving your body a healthy routine. You are not trying to punish it.

But with all the talk of workouts, is there something you can take to make the most out of your workout sessions?

It turns out there is.

The use of apple cider vinegar (ACV) is not something that arose recently. It has been used for thousands of years in cooking. Over the years, it began to gain popularity as a natural remedy for numerous disorders and ailments. In fact, just head over to your local store and you might just spot the number of apple cider vinegar brands that are now lining up the shelves. So why has this mixture gained a boost in popularity in recent years?

Here is one reason, the intake of the vinegar is considered to provide your body with plenty of benefits when combined with exercise including weight loss, lowered blood sugar levels, prevention of diabetes and more.

The best part of having apple cider vinegar is that it does not compromise on flavor. Many people have remarked on the fact that the vinegar is actually rather tasty.

So how can you combine ACV with your workouts? Is there anything else you should be adding to your intake of ACV?

Let us take an example. We have just discovered that ACV helps with weight loss. Imagine if you combine ACV with the Fat Removal Workout. You are not only going to enjoy the benefits of weight loss through your workout, but you are going to ensure that you manage your weight by consuming ACV.

While you are combining ACV with your exercises, you can add in another complimentary ingredient to the mix: creatine.

As you are engaged in managing your weight and creating a healthier lifestyle for yourself, you might need a source of energy for your workouts.

Why is creatine so useful? For one, it helps your muscles produce more energy. This means that you can work out without getting tired really fast. Additionally, creatine is a popular supplement for adding muscle mass. This means that you are not just maintaining a healthy routine, but you are improving your muscles as well.

Here are some of the other ways that creatine is useful for your body:

Supports High-Intensity Exercises

Creatine plays a vital role in the production of adenosine triphosphate, or ATP. Now, what is so special about this ATP? It actually does sound like the name of a medicinal drug. Thankfully, it isn't. However, it is an important component in your body. In fact, it is your body's energy source. When your body breaks down ATP, the process releases energy that is utilized by the tissues and various other parts of your body.

Fights Neurological Diseases

One of the reasons why neurological diseases spread really fast is because of the low levels of phosphocreatine in your brain. This reduces the energy levels supplied to your brain and weakens it. In research conducted on mice with Huntington's disease, adding creatine helped in restoring the brain's phosphocreatine levels. This improved brain functions and returned the brain to nearly 72% of its original state (or its pre-Huntington's disease state)! That is an incredible result and goes to show how just the absence one chemical can create such a drastic effect on the body. It also shows why creatine is not just a muscle booster. It is a powerful compound used for various processes in the body.

Brain Functions

As we are already focused on the region of the brain, let us continue to show how creatine further enhances the region. This is why meat is important.

Wait a minute. That was a random fact just throw in to show support to the meat eaters. Vegetarian for life!

That's not it. In fact, I wholly support a wholesome vegetarian meal. However, the fact remains and science backs it up:

meat is the best source of creatine. This is why vegetarians experience low levels of creatine in their bodies.

Does that mean you have to now give up your vegetarian diet and start sinking your teeth into some steak?! Not exactly. What you should be doing is adding creatine supplements to your diet to provide you with the necessary amount of the compound. In fact, in one study made on creatine, simply adding supplements that included the compound in the diet of vegetarians resulted in up to a 50% improvement in the intelligence and memory scores of the participants, showing an overall improvement in brain functions. Of course, if you are consuming meat, we are going to ensure that you consume the right meat as part of your OMAD diet. After all, what you eat plays a vital role in providing you with the right nutrients.

So imagine this scenario: you consume creatine to ensure that you have the energy for your exercises. You perform low- to moderate-intensity exercises to keep your body fit while you are dieting. You also add in ACV to ensure that you maintain your weight while throwing in some additional benefits such as prevention of diseases and lowering of your blood sugar levels. Sounds like a pretty potent combination, doesn't it?

And that is exactly why you should be adding creatine to your exercise routine along with a steady supply of ACV. It helps you maintain muscle while you are in a state of fasting.

Chapter 6: Foods You Think Are Keto-Friendly, But Aren't

We have all been there. We are certain that a particular food is definitely meant for our keto diet, only to discover that we have been wrong about that food. Trust me, I have encountered those scenarios quite a few times.

We are inundated with so much information that separating the wheat from the chaff becomes a challenging prospect. This becomes true when you have many sources of information claiming that they are backed up by science when they are in fact, just theories and guesses.

Most foods that you encounter in your life have carbs. Even certain types of meat, vegetables, and nuts contain some amount of carbs.

In fact, have you heard of the phrase "hidden carbs"?

You see, many dieters switch to low-carb diets each year. They are ready to give up a lot of foods such as bread, pasta, and rice. They decide to dial back on numerous fruits. They cut down on previous habits. Once all that is done, they believe that they are now of a journey to experience a low-carb diet! They have succeeded in creating the perfect plan for themselves!

Yet for all their efforts, they have no idea of some of the

sources of carbs. They might consume these foods, thinking that they are now safe within the boundaries of a low-carb diet.

If only they knew.

Here are some foods that actually have more carbs than you might have been aware of:

Low-Fat Foods

Have you ever walked by a supermarket aisle and spotted foods like dressings, peanut butter, and other items with the tag "low-fat"? Sounds tempting, doesn't it? It is like your prayers have been answered! Finally, you can enjoy some delicious food without worrying about any fattening ingredients.

Here is the reality of the situation. To ensure that the flavors of the low-fat products are not lost, food manufacturers generally replace fat with sugar. This increases the carb count rather than lowering it.

Liquid Eggs

In a world where you can get a canned or packaged version of so many foods (in fact, I actually spotted a pre-packed Indian butter chicken, how is that even possible?!), one of the ideas that has gained a fair amount of popularity in recent times is liquid eggs. You might have noticed containers of the stuff. All you have to do is pour them into a pan and you are ready to start cooking.

The reality? Not only do container eggs or liquid eggs contain certain ingredients and compounds that aren't usually found in an egg - such as xanthan gum – they are also infused with high fructose corn syrup (of course they are). Manufacturers are required to list the contents of their foods. But when you actually head over to products that contain corn syrup, you might notice something rather peculiar.

There is no mention of corn syrup on the label!

But how?!

Does this mean that you can now sue the company and win a million dollar lawsuit, after which you can finally retire on an island of your choice with a martini in your hand?! Quick, time to call in the best lawyers in the city!

Not so fast.

The reason why corn syrup is missing from the label is that it appears under another name: maltodextrin.

Pretty cunning isn't it?

Sauces

If your plate is covered with lots of healthy vegetables, then that is awesome! But if those vegetables are covered in a not-so-conservative amount of gravy and sauces, then you are about to consume a lot of carbs.

Restaurants need to sell their food. They need to make sure that the flavor is just right. Which is why, many of these outlets use sugar or flour, and both items contain a not-so-healthy dose of carbs. Before you know it, you are slurping away incredible amounts of carbs into your body. Yum!

Certain Vegetables

Oh yes. You might not have expected vegetables to turn up on this list but certain varieties of these foods actually contain a rather large amount of carbs. Brussel sprouts, broccoli, and squash are some examples that have high carbs but are still included in the diets of many people. This is because people are not actually aware of how many carbs these vegetables supply to you.

Want to know some of the other vegetables that are high in carbs?

Get ready because some of the items on this list might very well surprise you.

- Black-eyed peas

- Carrots

- Garbanzo beans

- Green peas
- Lima beans
- Parsnips
- Pinto beans
- Potato
- Pumpkin
- Sweet potato
- White beans

That is right. Carrots have high carbs too.

In fact, you might have been eating the vegetables in the above list and been confident of the fact that you are on the path to a healthy diet.

So what vegetables are actually safe to consume? Is there nothing that you can eat?

The answer is simple: you have a lot of options. In fact, you could be spoilt for choice when it comes to having vegetables with low-carbs. The trick is to identify them.

Spinach, mushroom, onion, asparagus, zucchini, eggplant, tomato, cabbage, peppers, and kale are just some of the examples of low-carb vegetables.

Once you begin to separate vegetables based on their carbs, you have a better idea of how you can manage your diet.

Chapter 7: 28 –Day OMAD Autophagy Meal Plan

There is a reason why OMAD works so well.

When you have one meal a day, you are storing fat only when you are feeding. This is because when you eat, insulin gets released into your bloodstream to regulate your blood sugar levels. Any extra sugar is then used for the muscles, liver, or stored as fat. When you are not eating, insulin does not get released and the aforementioned process does not occur.

If we actually start to think about it, the whole idea of having three or four meals a day does not sound practical. You are releasing insulin every time you eat. You are storing more and more fat in your body.

Nobody wants more fat.

Except perhaps your wallet. A fat wallet is a good sign.

But we are talking about your body so we are going to just use the required amount of fat.

And how do we do that?

We start with a 28-day OMAD Autophagy meal plan.

Remember, you are supposed to eat this meal anywhere between 5 pm to 7 pm.

Before we delve into some delicious recipes that you can enjoy during your OMAD diet, here are some important points that you should think about.

Caffeine

Caffeine is addictive and many of us consume way too much.

Most of us like to enjoy a nice cup of joe. That is okay. What is not okay is depending heavily on coffee to receive your energy. This is because our dependency becomes our weakness. We start taking too much of it and that ends up affecting our sleep patterns, which in turn begins to affect our fasting plan. When we drink coffee, we should aim to have a maximum of two cups a day. We should try not to have coffee beyond the 2 pm mark. Doing so might affect our sleep. While it is true that each person tolerates caffeine differently, it is not prudent to experiment just to get an extra cup of coffee in a day. Remember, you are heading towards a healthier lifestyle. Why ruin it?

Treats

Right, we all love to enjoy treats. And it becomes especially tempting to fall prey to your cravings when you are on a diet. But do not worry! I have included some incredible treats for you to enjoy. I also have a cappuccino treat waiting for you as well! So keep off those chocolate brownies for now.

Bread

People are so dependent on bread that they do not think twice about how many carbs they are consuming. It just becomes a natural part of their lives. In the following recipes, I have avoided bread to the best of my extent. Some people claim that having a single piece of bread occasionally is all right. Remember this, each person's body functions in a different way. You do not want to ruin your plan by trying to see if a single piece of bread will affect your body or not.

Sticking to the Schedule

I understand that people have commitments. You have to focus on different areas of your life and they might interrupt your OMAD plan. However, what is important to note is that there is no easy path to achieving good health. Want to gain weight? Pop some Cheetos and Nutella. Want to gain muscles? Sweat every day at the gym.

You see the difference there, right?

That is why I recommend that you try and stick to the plan as much as possible. It is true that the initial phase is going to be difficult. In fact, those who have ventured out to the gym know that the first few days involve quite a few muscle pains and cramps. Starting this diet will be no different.

The Grass Is Greener (and Healthier) on the

Other Side

Most people find the first week or so a challenging phase of the plan.

When your body begins to detox and cleanse, it may lead to headaches and lack of energy. You might decide that this plan is not worth it. But as I mentioned in the previous section, no matter what activity, course, plan, or sessions you choose to live a better life, you will always have to go through the tough introductory part.

There is, however, a way you can minimize some of the discomfort you might feel. Make sure you are rehydrating yourself with at least 2 liters of water.

Once you have passed the initial stages of the plan, the rest of the way is a walk in the park.

Note: As this is your only meal for the day, 4 "servings" is the serving size for 1 person. So your average calorie intake will be between 1600-1800 calories per day. If you require more (use this online tool to calculate your needs) https://www.active.com/fitness/calculators/bmr - then you can increase serving size as necessary.

Your OMAD Shopping List

Here are some of the things you should be shopping for when you hit the local supermarket. Do note that as you go through each recipe, you might get a better idea of the kind of ingredients that you might want to purchase.

Fats & Oils

Try to get your fat from natural sources like meat and nuts. Supplement with saturated and monounsaturated fats like coconut oil, butter, and olive oil.

Protein

Try to stick with organic, pasture-raised and grass-fed meat where possible. Most meats don't have added sugar in them, so they can be consumed in moderate quantity. Remember that too much protein on a ketogenic diet is not a good thing.

Vegetables

It does not matter whether you pick fresh or frozen vegetables. Stick with above ground vegetables, leaning toward leafy/green items.

Dairy

Most dairy is fine, but make sure to buy full-fat dairy items. Harder cheeses typically have fewer carbs.

Nuts and Seeds

In moderation, nuts and seeds can be used to create some fantastic textures. Try to use fattier nuts like macadamias and almonds.

Beverages

Stay simple and stick to mostly water. You can flavor it if needed with stevia-based flavorings or lemon/lime juice.

Day 1

Summer Shrimp Salad

Tomatoes, thyme, and shrimp make this not just a healthy meal but one that pleases the visual senses!

Serving Size

4 servings

Ingredients

1 ¼ pounds Raw Shrimps

3 large tomatoes (chopped)

1 medium-sized English cucumber

10 sprigs fresh thyme

¼ cup extra-virgin olive oil

4 cloves garlic (crushed)

¼ teaspoon salt

¼ teaspoon ground pepper

Thomas Hawthorn

¼ cup lemon juice

½ cup fresh basil (chopped)

Extra basil for garnish

Instructions

- Begin by preheating the oven to 350°F.

- Mix the shrimp with the thyme and garlic on a rimmed baking sheet. Add oil and mix again. Sprinkle the mixture with salt and pepper.

- Pop the mix into the oven and bake until you see the shrimp turning firm and pink: ideally for 8 – 10 minutes.

- Take out the mix and add your lemon juice. Stir the juice into the mix.

- Add in the tomatoes, cucumber, and basil and gently stir again.

- Next, transfer the salad into a bowl.

- Garnish it with basil to complete the meal prep.

Nutrition Information (per serving)

- Calories – 410 calories

- Fat – 15 grams

- Carbs – 8 grams

- Protein – 31 grams

Day 2

Grilled Fish Peperonata

Grilled fish with some peppers? Yes to the flavor please! If you like, you can prepare the peperonata in advance and then reheat it again when you are grilling the fish.

Serving Size

4 Servings

Ingredients

1 ½ pounds skinned swordfish, amberjack, or mahi-mahi

3 garlic cloves (sliced)

1 medium-sized red onion (thinly sliced)

8 cups bell peppers of any color (thinly sliced)

¼ cup fennel (thinly sliced)

1 teaspoon fresh oregano (chopped)

1 teaspoon fresh thyme (chopped)

1 teaspoon paprika

Thomas Hawthorn

½ teaspoon kosher salt

2 tablespoons sherry vinegar

2 tablespoons extra-virgin olive oil

Additional extra-virgin olive oil for grilling

Pinch of crushed red pepper

¼ cup parsley or basil for garnish

Instructions

- Heat 2 tablespoons of extra-virgin olive oil in a large pot over medium heat. Toss in your garlic, crushed red pepper, and cook. Stir occasionally (for about 2 to 3 minutes) until you can smell the fragrance and the garlic begins to show a brown color. Add the onion and continue stirring (for around 5 minutes) until the onions become soft.

- Add the oregano, paprika, and thyme.

- Add in the bell peppers and stir for around 10 seconds. Reduce the heat to a low degree and continue to cook the ingredients for about 15 to 20 minutes. Stir occasionally.

- Add the vinegar into the mix and cook for around 2 minutes more.

- Set the mixture aside and turn to the grill. Preheat the grill to a medium-high temperature. Use a brush and apply the oil to the fish, brushing gently. Sprinkle the fish with salt.

- Next, use the brush to oil the grill.

- Place the fish on the grill. Allow it to grill for around 5 minutes or until the flesh is opaque and then flip it over. Grill the other side for about 3 minutes or until you notice the opaque consistency.

- Take out the fish and use a cutting board to chop the fish into 4 pieces.

- Take out your plate. Place the peperonata on it (try and decorate your plate with it).

- Place your fish over the peperonata.

- Sprinkle with parsley or basil for garnish.

Nutrition Information (per serving)

- Calories – 420 calories

- Fat – 25 grams

- Carbs – 8.5 grams

- Protein – 32 grams

Day 3

Cuban Stromboli

A Cuban sandwich delight that adds the right amount of healthy ingredients and flavor! Plus, it has cheese.

Serving Size

6 servings

Ingredients

5 ounces pizza dough (whole wheat)

4 slices of Swiss cheese (preferably thin slices)

3 slices ham

3 slices turkey

4 slices salami

1 pickle sliced lengthwise

1 egg yolk (preferably large)

1 teaspoon water

Sesame seeds

Yellow mustard

Instructions

- Start off by preheating the oven to 450°F.

- Use a clean surface and lightly flour it. Roll out your pizza dough on the surface. Cut out rectangles measuring 12 inches by 6 inches.

- Add a layer of salami, ham, pickle, turkey, and Swiss cheese for each rectangular slice.

- Roll the slice along the long side of the rectangle. Ensure that the roll is tight.

- Take out your baking tray and cover it with a baking sheet.

- Place your rolls on the baking sheet.

- Use a knife to cut a few slits on the top of each roll.

- Take your egg yolk and add it to a bowl. Add the water into it. Whisk the mixture thoroughly.

- Use a brush to apply the yolk and water mixture on the top of the rolls.

- Sprinkle the rolls with sesame seeds.

- Pop the tray into the oven and bake it for not more than 20 minutes or until the rolls turn golden brown.

- Finally, serve the rolls with mustard if you like.

Nutrition Information (per serving)

- Calories – 276 calories

- Fat – 6 grams

- Carbs – 5 grams

- Protein – 4 grams

Day 4

Grilled Smoky Flank Steak

Who doesn't love a nice juicy steak? What? You thought this book was going to exclude steak? Not likely!

Serving Size

4 servings

Ingredients

5 pounds flank steak (trimmed)

1 ½ teaspoons smoked paprika

1 ½ teaspoons white vinegar

½ teaspoon ground chipotle chili

½ teaspoon salt

1 teaspoon brown sugar

¼ teaspoon ground pepper

¼ teaspoon garlic powder

Instructions

- Preheat your grill to a medium to medium-high temperature.

- In a small bowl, mix together the oil, chipotle chili, vinegar, garlic powder, paprika, salt, and pepper.

- One the ingredients are mixed well, use a brush and apply them over your steak. Alternatively, you can use your hands to rub the mixture over your steak. I prefer using your hands as it ensures that mixture is applied really well.

- Place your steak on the grill.

- Insert a thermometer into the thickest part of the steak.

- Grill until the thermometer reads about 120°F for a medium-rare steak.

- Once done, flip over the steak and grill again. Ideally, you should be grilling for 3 to 5 minutes per side.

- Take out the steak and place it on a plate. Allow it to rest for about 5 minutes

- Slice into 4 pieces.

Nutrition Information (per serving)

- Calories – 350 calories

- Fat – 12 grams

- Carbs – 2 grams

- Protein – 23 grams

Day 5

Crispy Salmon Caprese Salad

Another day, another exciting salad for you to eat. This time, we are jumping away from shrimp and entering the salmon territory.

Serving Size

4 servings

Ingredients

1 salmon fillet - large

1 cucumber (chopped) - large

1 cup cherry tomatoes (chopped in half)

1/2 cup fresh basil leaves (chopped)

4 tablespoons extra-virgin olive oil

1 tablespoon balsamic vinegar

½ teaspoon salt

½ teaspoon pepper

225 grams baby mozzarella balls

Instructions

- Let us get the salmon ready first. Take out a skillet and place it over medium-high heat. Allow it to heat up a little bit.

- Add 1 tablespoon of olive oil into the skillet. To spread the oil evenly, take out the skillet and gently rotate your wrist. Do not keep the skillet away from the flame for too long.

- Place the salmon skin side down into the skillet. Allow the salmon to cook for about 5 minutes. Turn over the salmon and cook the other side for about 3 to 4 minutes.

- Take out the salmon from the skillet. Remove the skin.

- In a large bowl, add tomatoes, cucumber, mozzarella balls, basil, and the remaining 3 tablespoons of olive oil. Mix well.

- Chop the salmon into small pieces and add them to the bowl. Mix again.

- Add salt and pepper to taste if you prefer. Add in the balsamic vinegar as well.

Nutrition Information (per serving)

- Calories – 407 calories

- Fat – 28 grams

- Carbs – 6 grams

- Protein – 29 grams

Day 6

Chicken Meatball Soup

A nice warm soup to add in a level of comfort after a hard day of fasting? Do I hear a "where do I get one?" Well, in your kitchen of course!

Serving Size

4 servings

Ingredients for the meatballs

2 chicken breasts, chopped

2 cloves garlic

2 tablespoon parsley (chopped)

1 tablespoon tomato puree

½ brown onion (chopped)

½ teaspoon salt

½ teaspoon pepper

1 tablespoon extra-virgin olive oil

Ingredients for the Soup

½ brown onion (chopped)

2 celery sticks, preferably medium (chopped)

2 carrots, preferably medium (chopped)

4 cups low-sodium chicken broth

1 teaspoon dried thyme

½ teaspoon salt

½ teaspoon pepper

1 tablespoon extra-virgin olive oil

Instructions

We'll start with the meatballs.

- Start by preheating the oven to 390°F.

- To make the meatballs, place all the ingredients for the meatballs inside a food processor and blitz them. Make sure that they appear well-combined.

- Begin creating rolls of meatballs, ideally with your hands.

- You should have no more than 20 meatballs, depending on the size.

- Take out a baking tray and cover it with a baking sheet.

- Take out a brush and apply the extra-virgin olive oil on the meatballs.

- Pop the tray into the oven and bake it for about 20 minutes or until you notice the meatballs turning a golden brown color.

While the meatballs are baking, time to prepare the soup.

- Take out a pan and heat at a medium-low setting. Add in the olive oil. Toss in the celery, onion, and carrots and stir them for about 4 to 5 minutes or until you see them softening.

- Add in the broth and the thyme. Season. Bring the soup to a boil and then reduce the heat to medium. Let the soup simmer for about 15 minutes.

- Add the kale into the soup and let cook for about 1 to 2

minutes or until it softens.

- Finally, add in your chicken meatballs.

Nutrition Information (per serving)

- Calories – 357 calories

- Fat – 19 grams

- Carbs – 6 grams

- Protein – 32 grams

Day 7

Green Shakshouka

Shakshouka is such a comfort food for many people. Turn it green with some spinach and feta and you have created a delicious and healthy meal to end your fast!

Serving Size

6 servings

Ingredients

12 ounces chard (stemmed properly and chopped)

12 ounces spinach (stemmed properly and chopped)

6 eggs, preferably large

Thomas Hawthorn

2 garlic cloves (chopped)

2 tablespoons unsalted butter

1 onion (chopped), preferably large

1 small serrano pepper (thinly sliced)

½ cup low-sodium chicken broth

½ cup feta cheese

4 tablespoons extra-virgin olive oil

1 tablespoon balsamic vinegar

¼ teaspoon salt

¼ teaspoon pepper

Instructions

- Place a skillet over medium heat. Allow it to heat up a little.

- Once the skillet is hot, add in the oil and allow it to heat as well.

- Add in the onion and begin cooking. Stir in as frequently as possible for about 7 to 8 minutes, until you begin to notice the onions turning translucent and soft. However, do not allow the onions to brown.

- Add the spinach and the chard into the skillet. The best

way to add them is by handfuls. Take a handful of chard and spinach, place it into the skillet and then repeat the process. Cook them until you notice them becoming wilted, which typically happens in about 5 minutes.

- Add in your balsamic vinegar, serrano, garlic, salt, and pepper. Stir the ingredients together for about 2 to 4 minutes until you notice the garlic softening.

- Bring in the broth and the butter to the mixture. Continue stirring until the butter melts.

- Next, take your eggs and crack them over the vegetables.

- Place a cover over the skillet and then turn the heat to medium-low. Cook the shakshouka for about 3 to 5 minutes until you see the eggs turn white.

- Finally, remove the skillet from heat and sprinkle it with cheese. Place the cover over the skillet again and allow it to rest for about 2 minutes before serving.

Nutrition Information (per serving)

- Calories – 296 calories

- Fat – 23 grams

- Carbs – 5 grams

- Protein – 11 grams

Day 8

Crispy Artichokes

Imagine this, delicious crispy artichokes placed on top of smooth labneh. Boy that is one way to sit down, relax, and enjoy a meal that just brings a smile to your face. You might have to start preparing the recipe in the morning or at least a week in advance as a part of the recipe relies on refrigeration. I would recommend that you start a week in advance.

Serving Size

6 servings

Ingredients

4 cups plain yogurt. I highly recommend the whole-milk variety. Other forms of yogurt have high carbs.

4 cups canola oil

4 cloves garlic

3 tablespoons lemon juice

2 cans of artichoke hearts. Make sure you rinse them, then halve them, and finally set them out to dry

¼ cup parsley (chopped)

Instructions

- Firstly, you will need a sieve and a bowl. The bowl should be deep enough that if you place the sieve inside the bowl, there are at least 3 inches of space between the bottom of the sieve and the bowl. Ensure that the sieve has a diameter of at least 7 inches or bigger.

- Next, place 4 layers of cheesecloth into the sieve. Make sure that you line each cheesecloth properly. Then place the sieve into the bowl.

- In another bowl, add the yogurt and pour the lemon juice into it. Whisk them well. Transfer the yogurt mixture from the second bowl into the sieve. Make sure that you get as much of the yogurt into the sieve as possible.

- Now you have to refrigerate until the yogurt is thick and you notice at least 1 cup of liquid has drained into the bowl. As mentioned earlier, you can choose to refrigerate it starting early in the morning or up to 1 week in advance.

- Once you have refrigerated the labneh for the recommended duration, take out the sieve and discard the liquid.

- Transfer the sieve into a medium bowl.

- Add ¼ tablespoon of salt and stir well.

- Now it is time to work on the artichokes. Pour the oil into a large saucepan and bring it to medium-high heat. Start frying your artichokes for about 2 to 3 minutes until they turn golden brown and crispy.

- Transfer the artichokes to a medium-sized bowl (yes, this recipe is going to require quite a few bowls). Add in the garlic, parsley, and the remaining salt.

- Finally, take the labneh and spread it over a plate. Add the crispy artichokes on top.

- If you prefer, you can serve the dishes with a couple of lemon wedges.

Nutrition Information (per serving)

- Calories – 323 calories

- Fat – 26 grams

- Carbs – 13 grams

- Protein – 10 grams

Day 9

Bacon with Sautéed Radishes

We had steak. Now it is time to introduce some bacon into your diet. One of the best aspects of this dish is that it is easy to make and even if you do not like radishes, you might just find them enjoyable after this meal.

Serving Size

4 servings

Ingredients

12 ounces radishes (quartered)

6 shallots (quartered), preferably medium

3 slices bacon (chopped)

2 teaspoons garlic (finely chopped)

1 teaspoon fresh thyme (chopped)

1 ½ tablespoons cider vinegar

1 ½ teaspoons unsalted butter

¼ teaspoon salt

¼ teaspoon pepper

Instructions

- Place a skillet over medium-high heat.

- Once the skillet is hot, place the bacon strips into the skillet. Flip the bacon occasionally for about 5 to 6 minutes until they turn crispy.

- Cover a plate with a paper towel. Transfer the bacon onto the plate. Make sure that you leave the drippings in the skillet.

- Add in the shallots and the radishes. Cook them for about 2 to 3 minutes until they are charred slightly on one side. Once you notice the char, continue to cook until they turn brown all over. Make sure you do not char them too much at this point.

- Throw in your thyme and garlic and stir.

- Add the salt and pepper and continue to stir for about 1 minute until you smell the fragrance.

- Take the skillet off the heat and then add in the butter and vinegar.

- Mix everything together well.

- Finally, add the thyme as a garnish.

Nutrition Information (per serving)

- Calories – 285 calories

- Fat – 12 grams

- Carbs – 9 grams

- Protein – 5 grams

Day 10

Cappuccino Chia Macadamia Pudding

When you deserve to enjoy a nice treat, you can simply make this little delight. Did I also mention that it is actually healthy?

Serving Size

6 servings

Ingredients

1 cup chia seeds

½ cup espresso

3 cups and 3 tablespoons macadamia or almond milk (make sure you get the unsweetened variety)

1 teaspoon vanilla extract (sugar-free)

1 teaspoon cacao powder or cinnamon

Stevia to taste

Instructions

Starting with the coffee

Thomas Hawthorn

- Add ⅔ cup of chia seeds to a blender and grind them into a powder (alternately, keep the seeds whole for more texture).

- Next, pour in 2 cups and 2 tablespoons of your macadamia or almond milk as well as the ½ cup of espresso.

- Blend it all together and taste, add stevia if desired.

- Pour into your cup till the cup is ⅔ full and cool the mix in the fridge.

Continuing with the vanilla topping

- Clean the blender then add in ⅓ cup chia seeds, the remaining 1 cup and 1 tablespoon of macadamia or almond milk, 1 teaspoon vanilla extract, 1 teaspoon of cacao powder. Blend until smooth.

- Add stevia to taste, if desired.

- Pour this on top of the coffee and cool in the fridge for at least an hour prior to serving.

- You can sprinkle additional cacao powder on top right before serving to give it some extra flavor.

Nutrition Information (per serving)

- Calories – 151 calories

- Fat – 9.7 grams

- Carbs – 2.4 grams

- Protein – 5.8 grams

Day 11

Tomato Dolma

Time to have a few stuffed vegetables. Especially if the stuffing is ground beef and eggplants.

Serving Size

12 servings

Ingredients

12 tomatoes, preferably medium sized

3 tablespoons bulgur

2 tablespoons extra-virgin olive oil

2 cloves garlic

1 eggplant, preferably large

1 onion, preferably medium

1 teaspoon ground cumin

1 pound ground beef

Thomas Hawthorn

1 teaspoon salt

½ teaspoon pepper

¼ cup fresh mint (chopped)

Instructions

- Start off by preheating the grill on high heat.

- Next, use a fork to prick an eggplant. Now slowly grill it, making sure you turn occasionally. Grill for 10 to 15 minutes until you notice the eggplant turn tender and charred. Transfer to a plate to cool. Once cool, peel the eggplant and transfer it to a bowl. Add the juices from the plate into the bowl and mash the eggplant. Let it sit for 10 minutes.

- Next, preheat your oven to 400°F. Take out a baking dish and lightly coat it with cooking spray.

- Take your tomatoes and cut off their tops. Do not dispose of the tops as we will require them later. Remove the inside of the tomato with a spoon.

- Take the insides of the tomato and place them in a blender. Add oil, ¼ teaspoon salt, and pepper and then blend it until it becomes a puree. Take the puree and spread it inside the baking dish.

- Use some of the remaining salt to sprinkle the insides

of the tomatoes.

- Return to the eggplant. Add the ground beef, garlic, onion, bulgur, cumin, and the remaining salt and pepper into the eggplant. Mix well. Take the mixture and stuff the tomatoes with it.

- Replace the cut-off tops of the tomatoes.

- Place the tomatoes in the baking dish, use foil to cover the dish.

- Place the dish in the oven and bake for about 15 minutes. Next, take off the foil and continue baking for another 30 or 35 minutes.

- Take out the dish and sprinkle the tomatoes with mint.

Nutrition Information (per serving)

- Calories – 131 calories

- Fat – 9 grams

- Carbs – 3 grams

- Protein – 9 grams

Day 12

Thomas Hawthorn

Low-Carb Walnut and Zucchini Salad

Walnut and zucchini are both healthy foods. Combine them and you have a healthy salad to finish your day.

Serving Size

4 servings

Ingredients for the Dressing

2 tablespoons olive oil

2 teaspoons lemon juice

1 garlic clove

¼ cup low-carb mayonnaise

½ teaspoon salt

¼ teaspoon chili powder

Ingredients for the Salad

4 ounces arugula lettuce

2 zucchini

1 head of Romaine lettuce

1 tablespoon olive oil

¾ cup chopped walnuts or pecans

¼ cup finely chopped fresh chives or scallions

¼ teaspoon salt

¼ teaspoon pepper

Instructions

- Take out a small bowl. Toss in all the ingredients necessary to make the dressing and whisk them together well. Set aside the dressing so that the flavors develop. In the meantime, turn your attention to the salad.

- Cut the zucchini into halves length-wise and remove the seeds. Next, chop the zucchini halves, preferably into half-inch pieces.

- Take out a frying pan and pour the olive oil in it. Allow the oil to heat up over medium heat until you see it simmering.

- Place your chopped zucchini in the pan. Season it with salt and pepper.

- Sauté the zucchini until it turns a light brown color.

- Trim and cut the salad. Place the romaine, arugula, and chives in a large bowl.

- Next, cut the lettuces and mix them into the large

bowl.

- Add in your zucchini and mix well.

- Take out your nuts and roast them in the same pan you used to prepare your zucchini. Season lightly with salt and pepper.

- Toss them into the bowl with the zucchini and mix well.

- Finally, drizzle your salad with the dressing.

Nutrition Information (per serving)

- Calories – 456 calories

- Fat – 54 grams

- Carbs – 7 grams

- Protein – 8 grams

Day 13

Low-carb Tartlets with Caramelized Onion and Brie

These little delights remind you of mini pies, minus all the carbs and calories!

Serving Size

12 tartlets

Ingredients for the Crust

1 batch of keto pie crust

Ingredients for the Cheese filling

2 medium red onions (thinly sliced)

2 tablespoons extra-virgin olive oil

2 tablespoons balsamic vinegar (30 ml)

12 small wedges brie cheese

¼ cup fresh herbs such as thyme or rosemary

½ teaspoon sea salt, for taste

Instructions

- Preheat the oven to 355°F.

- Next, take out a frying pan and place it over medium heat. Pour a little olive oil into it and bring it to a simmer.

- Toss in your onions, and cook. Stir occasionally until you see the onions soften.

- Bring down the heat to low. Add your vinegar and salt,

and continue cooking. Stir occasionally. Wait until the onions have caramelized.

- While the onions are becoming caramelized, take out 12 muffin tins. Grease them inside and press your pie crust into these muffin tins.

- Once done, pop them into the oven and bake for about 10 minutes. Remove the pie crusts from the oven and allow them to cool at room temperature, ideally for about 5 minutes.

- Once the crusts have cooled slightly, take out the onions and divide them equally among the tart cases.

- Cut the brie into 12 even pieces and place them atop the onions. Sprinkle some herbs on them for garnish.

- Put the crusts back into the oven and bake them for about 15 minutes, until you notice the tops getting brown.

- As soon as they brown, take them out of the oven and serve.

- You can even keep the tartlets refrigerated and have them the next day.

Nutrition Information (per serving)

- Calories – 220 calories

- Fat – 12 grams

- Carbs – 2 grams

- Protein – 10 grams

Day 14

Low-Carb Veggie Fritters

These crispy delights are packed with some incredible nutrients. Typically, they are made using unsalted butter. However, as we would like to increase the fat content, we are going to make use of ghee. Whatever you choose, however, the result is delicious and crispy fritters.

Serving Size

12 fritters

Ingredients

4 medium eggs

1 zucchini, preferably large and grated

1 carrot, preferably medium and grated

½ celeriac, preferably medium and grated

1 cup sauerkraut (drained)

1 yellow onion, small and diced

½ teaspoon sea salt

½ teaspoon chili flakes, for flavor

2 tablespoons ghee or duck fat, for cooking

Instructions

- Pour water in a bowl. Add in the celeriac and carrots. Add the salt into the mixture. Stir and set it aside for about 15 minutes.

- Take another bowl and place a muslin cloth in it. Transfer your celeriac and carrots to the bowl.

- Add the zucchini and the sauerkraut.

- Next, squeeze out the water and any juices. Discard the liquid.

- Place the vegetables into a bowl once they are drained and mix them with eggs. Add your chili flakes for seasoning if you prefer.

- Place a pan over medium-low heat. Pour your ghee into the pan. Fry for about 5 or 6 minutes.

- Next, flip the fritters over and fry them on the other side for another 5 or 6 minutes.

- Repeat the process if needed until the fritters are cooked well.

Nutrition Information (per serving)

- Calories – 223 calories

- Fat – 11 grams

- Carbs – 5 grams

- Protein – 6 grams

We have reached halfway through your daily meal plan. At this point, you should be well acclimated to the new type of diet as you have already been incorporating it into your life for two weeks. You might not struggle with the diet as much as you did in the beginning.

Day 15 - 28

For the remaining days, you can simply combine what you have prepared during the first 14 days or repeat the diet all over again. One tip that you can follow is to start preparing your meals in the reverse order that you had prepared them for the first 14 days.

The choice is entirely yours.

24, 48, and 72-hour Fasts. Are They Even Possible?

Yes, they are.

Most people think of fasting for such long periods as completely crazy! How can you go 24 hours or more without food? And why would you do it?!

Many reasons.

Perhaps you might be traveling to another country and the airport or plane food might not suit your body (it is fairly common for many people). You might not want to resort to the plane food just because you are hungry. Oftentimes, it also depends on the plane you are traveling in. If you have chosen a low-budget airline, then you might not have complete faith in their food quality. Whatever your reasons are, you could use a 24-hour fast to make sure that you skip any unsuitable food until you reach a place where you can finally dig in to some good stuff.

In many cases, people might find the local food in the country they are visiting unsuitable for them. Let us suppose that you are traveling to Thailand for a business trip for about 48 hours. Let us also assume that Thai food and your stomach are not exactly BFFs. Instead of forcing yourself to eat the local food, you could fast until you are back home.

These are just some examples of why people would prefer to go fasting.

Of course, we cannot discount the most important factor: the cleansing of your body.

So how do you prepare yourself for each of the fasting periods mentioned above?

24 hour fast

The first thing that you should do is put your body into a state of ketosis. If you have been following our meal plan or if you have gotten started on it, then you have practically completed your initiation into ketosis.

On the morning of the day of the fast, drink a cup of water with a little sea salt added to it. This will replace the electrolytes in your body. It also helps lower cortisol levels which will help to reduce your stress. You see, you should aim to keep your stress levels low in the morning.

Additionally, make sure you get a good night's rest before you start the day of fasting. If you are sleep deprived, then your blood sugar levels increase and it enters into your kidneys. This causes you to urinate frequently, which in turn causes you to get thirsty really fast.

Once you have your water in the morning, you then have to wait for about two to three hours before you can consume coffee or tea, should you choose to. However, you need to make sure that you are having black coffee or plain tea only. No milk. No sugar.

During your fast, what you can also do, and which I recommend that you do, is drink mineral water. But make sure you do not drink too much of it as it could cause frequent urination.

What do you do if you do feel hungry? One of the important things to remember is that when you are in a state of ketosis you do not feel hungry because your body is deprived of essential nutrients. You feel hungry at specific times because your body has been trained to receive food during those times. In other words, your body is on autopilot and reacts to the circadian rhythm that you have set up for yourself. It is time for you to take back control of your appetite. To curb your hunger, you can drink coffee (black only). Coffee is one of the best appetite suppressants. It also promotes the production of ketone bodies in your body.

Do not consume artificial sweeteners. Despite what you hear about them, they are known to cause an insulin response in your body. Which is why it is preferable to stay away from them.

Make sure that you are also engaged in low-intensity exercises. These help you deplete liver glycogen, which eventually helps promote ketosis even more.

48 hour fast

A 48-hour fast might be difficult for beginners. I strongly recommend working on the 24-hour fast before you try out this fast. What you are doing here is trying to remain on a water diet for a 48-hour period. The primary purpose of this fast is to cleanse your body and give it an opportunity to heal. According to doctors who have looked into the water diet during a long fast, the water fast encourages rapid regeneration of the intestine's mucosal lining. This type of fasting also gives cells the ability to eliminate waste and rid the body of harmful toxins.

The best way to go about this type of fast is by getting into OMAD. Once you are comfortable around it, then you are ready to fast for a 48-hour period.

Let us assume that your last OMAD meal was at 7 pm. Your next course of action would be to head to bed and get a good night's sleep.

The next day, you are going to drink mineral water or water with sea salt in the morning to replenish your electrolytes.

During the afternoon, you can have your cup of coffee to reduce the feeling of hunger. For the rest of the day, you should drink mineral water frequently.

When you reach the evening, you might feel a pang of hunger. At this time, you simply have to take a glass of water and add one or two teaspoons of apple cider vinegar into it. ACV has practically zero calories. But what it also has is potassium and magnesium which replenishes the electrolytes in your body and help stave off hunger.

The first 24 hours of your fast is the most challenging time. Think of it like cresting a hill. The first 24 hours are like going uphill. You will feel the challenge. However, once you cross the top (the 24-hour mark), it is all a smooth downhill experience from there.

Finally, you should be having your final OMAD meal once you complete the fast.

72 hour fast

This is one of the most challenging fasts you will experience and I would highly recommend starting out with the 24-hour fast before you even think of venturing into the 72-hour fast.

Apart from that, there are a few protocols that you can follow before you begin your 72-hour fast.

The first being that you should be on your OMAD diet for at least three to five days. When you are on your OMAD diet, you are going to be significantly less hungry during the fasting period. Your body is going to produce ketones. It will cleanse itself of bad cells and proteins. It is starting to use good fats as its fuel source rather than carbs. In short, it will prepare you for the fast.

The second protocol that you should be following is loading your body with water and sodium. To find sodium in water, you should always opt for mineral water. As we saw before, your body tends to urinate when it has less sodium. Now, urinating itself is not a bad process. This is because you drop all those harmful substances that your body possesses. However, urination means that the water content in your body is slightly dipping. This means that you have to supplement the water lost during the process. Another question that you might ask is why sodium is vital to the body. The main reason is that sodium helps maintain the fluids in your body in a normal state, such as your body water. This means that you do not feel dehydrated quickly.

Another reason why sodium is important is that when your body has a lack of the substance, then you activate certain receptors in your body called NST receptors. These receptors send signals to your brain that you need to have food. More specifically, it craves foods with salt content, as salt contains high amounts of sodium. This means you start getting hungry really fast.

Once you have the above protocols set into place, you can practically ease your way into a long-term fast. It becomes easier and you do not feel the strong effects of hunger while you are fasting.

When you are fasting, make sure that you are consuming the

Thomas Hawthorn

below items only:

Water (mineral, tap or sparkling)

Coffee

Apple Cider Vinegar

Tea

When it comes to the kind of tea you are consuming, make sure you take in only green tea. This is because green tea has epigallocatechin gallate, or EGCG. One of the most important functions of the EGCG is that it helps our body activate certain enzymes and genetic processes that help us during our fast. You feel more in control of your appetite.

Another important component of green tea is theanine. This important ingredient of tea helps your body produce more gamma-aminobutyric acid. This acid helps you remain calmer and satiate you during your fast.

Why is remaining calm essential? Any time you get anxious, stressed, or experience negative mental states, your body releases higher amounts of cortisol. This hormone increases the insulin levels in your body. Your sugar levels then drop and you eventually become hungry.

Finally, get plenty of rest. Do not skip out on a good night's sleep. You do not want to stress your body, either physically or mentally.

With these tips in mind, you are ready to begin an incredible and rejuvenating fasting experience.

Chapter 8: Keto Autophagy Lifestyle

You have now entered the OMAD lifestyle. It has its ups and downs, but you are finding yourself able to manage your fast so far. You feel confident about the fast and of your capability to deal with it.

Is there anything else that you need to consider?

There is.

You see, getting used to the fast is just one side of the coin, you need to maintain the lifestyle as well.

Here are a few tips to enjoy a comfortable and rewarding keto autophagy experience.

Stay Hydrated

This is a no brainer. We have already seen how hydration helps with your fast. You need to ensure that you refill your body's water levels. As your kidneys produce urine, you expunge your body of harmful materials. That in itself is not a bad thing. Urinating is one of the ways your body gets rid of waste. However, when you urinate, your body water levels become irregular and you can lower the levels of water and sodium in your body. This means that you need to replenish the water levels of your body.

Eat Your Meals Slowly

This is different from chewing your food many times. Often, people tend to gobble down their food quickly. When you eat slowly, you help your body digest food more effectively. You also lose weight more quickly and without much discomfort. At the same time, you feel satiated with each meal you have. What you are doing by eating slowly is that you are giving your body the time to extract the nutrients from each bite you take. That means you feel more satisfied with your meal.

When you eat fast, you tend to push down your portion. Which is why many people still feel hungry even after having a rather fulfilling meal. If you rush through your food you affect your digestion. Your meals become a stressful situation. Your body might send signals indicating that the meal was over too soon and it probably means that you did not have enough. Add to that the fact that sometimes the stress your body endures gets translated to a rise in cortisol. We do not want that happening.

Improve Your Sleep Patterns

If you are not having proper sleep, then your body will automatically elevate its levels of stress hormones. This leads to irregular blood sugar levels. I recommend that you head to bed before 11 pm. Ensure that you are sleeping in a dark room. Keep mobile phones and other devices away from you as radiation from these devices can affect your sleep. Make sure you are not using these devices for at least an hour before you sleep. I also recommend getting 7 to 9 hours of good sleep each night.

How to Adapt to OMAD

Societal Pressure

Just take a look around you. There is no shortage of foods available. There are stores at nearly every corner of your area. You have vending machines providing you quick snacks. Your refrigerator, kitchen, and probably even your room might be filled with options that could tempt you out of a keto diet.

However, these temptations can be managed.

What you might find difficult to manage is the pressure you receive from society. You see, most people are not used to taking up a keto diet. It becomes rather difficult for them or they give up too easily. Others simply choose to not believe in the diet, thinking that it is simply an absurd idea concocted by someone to make a lot of money.

But the reality is that in today's world, people are becoming more aware. They want to focus on something that is backed by science, practice, and results. When the keto diet entered the scene, there were a lot of skeptics. Is this another way to bamboozle us out of our money? Am I going to do something that does not generate any result?

Over time, science decided to jump in on the subject of keto dieting. Scientists and society wanted to know whether the diet actually works. As more and more facts began to pile up, researchers realized that the keto diet is not based on a random collection of facts.

It is a scientifically studied method.

But even so, you might feel compelled to shift away from the diet because the people around you might convince you to do so. Or you might look at others enjoying all the meals in the world and it might make you wonder if it's worth taking on the keto diet.

Let me tell you that people have found results through ketogenic autophagy and OMAD routines.

I am not just referring to physical changes. I am talking about improving your focus, attention, memory, and productivity. I am talking about longevity. Because keto does not simply throw in a process for the sake of doing so. A keto diet focuses on certain aspects of our life and chooses to enhance those areas.

So do not worry about what others say. You are on a path to bring a healthy change into your life. And while it may be a difficult path (when is progress not difficult?) there is a big reward at the end of the journey.

Thomas Hawthorn

Hunger Levels

You are going to feel the discomfort of hunger when you begin your OMAD journey. After all, you are plunging yourself into a new lifestyle after decades of sticking to specific routines, patterns, and indulgences.

It takes time to adjust.

However, there are many ways you can deal with hunger while you are on your OMAD diet. I have already shown you steps to work on your hunger while you are in the middle of a 24, 48, or 72-hour diet. You can apply the same steps to manage hunger during OMAD.

Remember that the key to a successful one meal a day plan lies in your willpower. Sure, it is challenging to go through a diet plan. However, the challenge becomes manageable when you realize that your body is not the one demanding food, your brain is.

Your body has all the nutrients it requires. Unfortunately, your brain is used to decades of conditioning and is refusing to let go of its old belief systems and habits.

When you master your mind, you can master your body.

That notion becomes true when you are going through OMAD.

Breaking Fast: How to Break Fast the Right Way

When you are ready to break your fast your body is primed to take in the nutrients that you provide. It's like a vacuum, switch it on and whoosh! In goes your food faster than you can spell the word "digest".

This means that it is ready to absorb all those nutrients quickly. While you may think that your stomach working really fast means that you get more nutrients into your body, then that is not true. Remember our section on eating slowly? There is a reason we included that. We are aiming for your digestive processes to take in all the nutrients without sending any of them to the waste bin.

In a similar way, do not break your fast by eating something.

Get your body ready. Let it know that there is awesome stuff incoming.

To get your body into a state of readiness, try the below techniques:

Drink ACV, Lemon Water, or Bone Broth

We had already established that ACV is not just vital for your body during fasting but it also helps you gain some extra elements vital for you.

Lemon water is known to improve digestion. This is why having it before your meal preps your body to work on your food more effectively.

Similarly, bone broth plays a vital role in promoting digestive health.

There really is no better or worse option. Simply choose the drink that you prefer and have it before you begin to break your fast.

For Muslims, the month of Ramadan is a holy month. It involves the process of fasting from dawn till dusk as part of their mandatory ritual. Ramadan occurs every year and Muslims prepare their body for the fast in many ways.

What is important to note is the routine they follow during the fasting process. You see, when it comes time to break their fast, they do not immediately sit down to eat. They most commonly consume dates and follow that with a glass of water.

They are preparing their body for receiving food.

Of course, we are not going to eat dates because the fruit has high sugar content.

However, the concept of breaking your fast by preparing your body in advance is still a vital component of Muslim fasting.

What we are doing is fairly similar, minus all the high carb and high sugar foods.

To successfully break your fast, make sure you take in a glass of water with two teaspoons of ACV, a glass of lemon water, or bone broth 30 minutes to around 1 hour before you plan to eat a solid meal.

Supplementary Support

Taking supplements can help you with your fasting. They not only help you manage your hunger, but they infuse your body with essential nutrients. Let us examine some of the supplements that you can take during OMAD and the kind of benefits they provide your body.

Vitamin D3

If you would like your body to absorb more calcium and improve the growth of your bones, then you need vitamin D3. When you have little of the substance in your body, your bones could turn fragile or, in some cases, misshapen. Adding a little vitamin D during your fast helps you sustain yourself better during the fast.

Vitamin D plays an important role in the maintenance of calcium and phosphorus levels in the blood. These two compounds influence the way your bones develop tremendously.

Additionally, we also need vitamin D to absorb calcium in the intestines and to ensure that too much calcium does not get excreted through the kidneys.

Thomas Hawthorn

Fish Oil

In the past decade, many health physicians and doctors have recommended fish oil to their patients. But what makes this supplement so popular?

For one, fish oil contains omega-3 fatty acids. These are helpful for the following reasons:

- Reduce blood pressure

- Lower the instances of your heart picking up an abnormal rhythm

- Lower the chances of strokes and heart attacks

Fish oil becomes especially important when you are working out. Combine all of the above benefits and the fact that fish oil reduces muscle soreness and joint pains, then you have the ideal supplement to take for your workouts.

L-Carnitine

L-Carnitine is an amino acid that is naturally produced in your body. As you grow older, your body reduces the supply of L-Carnitine. This causes your body to slow down, have reduced energy, and prevents you from enjoying an active lifestyle. As your activity reduces, you easily gain weight. When you are fasting, you should aim to be as active as possible. In order to help you with that, you can take L-Carnitine as a supplement. The amino acid becomes especially useful when you are about to workout, giving you a quick boost of energy for your exercises.

Do note that the best time to take the supplement would be first thing in the morning and on an empty stomach. You could also take it later during the day, but make sure you are taking it at least 30 minutes before you break your fast.

Turmeric

Turmeric is a popular spice in India. In fact, many of the dishes in the country include turmeric as a vital ingredient. If you've ever wondered how Indian curries gain their yellow color, then you now know the answer why. Yes indeed, it is turmeric.

Indians consider turmeric as having medicinal properties.

In wasn't until recently that science has started to understand why Indians believe that turmeric provides them with health benefits. One of the most important components of turmeric is curcumin. Why is this component vital? Curcumin is what gives turmeric its anti-inflammatory properties. It is also a strong anti-oxidant. Which is why, you can choose to add turmeric either into your food, or you can have supplements made out of turmeric. Either way, you are making sure that your body receives the right amount of curcumin.

Exercising During Fasting

When you exercise during your OMAD diet, you are forcing your body to remove fat. This is because the process of burning fats in your body is managed by your sympathetic nervous system (SNS). Why is this important? Well, one of the major ways in which you can activate your SNS is by exercising and lack of food.

This is why numerous health and fitness experts recommend including exercises as part of your fasting regime. As we saw before, resistance training can be incorporated into your diet.

Remember the following tips before you start performing your exercises and while you are exercising:

Always warm up before you dive into any exercise.

Stick to a routine that is comfortable for you. Do not overdo it.

Focus on using the right form and posture. Do not think about momentum. You might have noticed people in the gym using momentum and showing how they are exerting a lot of energy. This is not always because they are working really hard. Sometimes, it is because they are performing the wrong posture and that tends to force people to add more energy than is necessary.

Chapter 9: What to Do if Your Weight Loss Plateaus

You have now been following a strict diet. You have been working hard to maintain a healthy OMAD diet and improve your exercise routines. You can see progress. Your reward for exercising has been seeing your weight go down and your overall health improve. All of a sudden and for no reason you can understand, the weight on the scale has stopped decreasing. What the heck?! Did you do something wrong?! Has the diet stopped working?

Fear not, my friend. You have only reached a point that every individual who goes on a diet reaches. You have reached a weight-loss plateau.

Do not feel disheartened. There is nothing to worry about. It is completely normal for weight loss to slow down a bit and sometimes even just remain at a particular point for a while.

When you begin to understand the mechanisms behind a weight-loss plateau, you have the power to know how to react and prevent giving up on your OMAD diet.

During the initial period of your weight-loss regime, you might notice a rapid drop in your weight. You might feel a sense of exhilaration.

This drop happens because when you curb down your

calories, your body gets the necessary energy by releasing its reserves of glycogen. Glycogen is a type of carbohydrate that is found in the liver and the muscles.

Glycogen contains water. This is why, when glycogen is used by the body for energy, it releases water. This water release causes your weight to plummet down like a skydiver in freefall.

When you see the rapid drop in weight, it is definitely a wonderful moment. However, it is a temporary situation.

As you continue to lose weight, you also some muscles as well. Here is the thing about muscles, they help you maintain the rate at which calories are burnt in your body. In other words, they manage the speed of your metabolism. This is why, the more weight you lose, the more muscles are lost. This causes your metabolism to lower, leading to a decrease in the rate of burning calories. Eventually, the rate at which you lose weight declines.

At this point, your metabolism has slowed down. But it does not stop entirely. This is why you are still losing weight, just not at the same rate as before. Eventually, you reach a point where you are consuming the same amount of calories as you burn.

That is when your weight loss plateaus.

Additionally, because our bodies have ways to increase our

resilience and longevity during times of fasting, our brains will trigger a variety of mechanisms to keep us from losing more weight. Why does this happen?

Evolution.

Back when our ancestors were hunting for food, they often faced situations of famine. They had no technology to protect them during those times and starvation was a common problem. In fact, some of the mass exoduses in human history were made to avoid famine and find better places for food. But I digress. Back to our bodies.

As time went on, our bodies evolved to protect us during times of famine. It did not want us to lose more weight because weight loss meant getting weaker. And if people got weaker, then that meant they were next in line to be on the buffet menu of a saber-tooth tiger.

No one likes to be on the menu of a saber-tooth tiger.

Nowadays, there are no sabretooth tigers. But that does not mean that our evolutionary traits have been expunged from our bodies. They still exist.

So when you enter a state of fasting, your brain thinks it is experiencing famine. That's when it activates mechanisms to prevent weight loss.

As you can see, nothing to worry about. Not even saber-tooth tigers.

To begin losing weight, all you need to do is either have more physical activity on a daily basis or reduce the calories you eat. Thankfully for us, OMAD means you increase activities and decrease calories. You are getting the best of both worlds. When you use the same level of physical activity that you had before you began your diet, then you may not lose too much weight.

Track Your Calories. Recalculate Your Macros.

To count or not to count, that is an interesting question. When you are losing calories, you might feel conflicted about measuring your calories. On one hand, you may not want to see how your progress is going on. Will you be surprised? Will you be disappointed? Questions like that make you hesitant about checking your calories. When you maintain a record or keep a track of the calories you consume from your meals, you encourage yourself to make better choices. You become responsible for the changes happening to your body. You are now accountable for the results that occur because of your dieting. Moreover, you can keep a constant check on your progress.

You can use this online tool to calculate your macros https://www.active.com/fitness/calculators/bmr

Whether you receive good news or bad news, you should have

a sense of awareness about what is happening to your body. Do not fool yourself into thinking that something is happening. Be certain. Be informed. You see, you cannot fool yourself with arbitrary numbers and statistics when you jot down your calorie count. Recording your food consumption and knowing what you eat is an important part of losing weight. It is better to eat a wonderful salad than to waste time-consuming a nutritious meal that may not even be working out for you.

Your choices matter. Make informed ones.

This is why your decisions matter when you realize that your weight plateaus. Imagine working so hard but not realizing that nothing is happening to your body. Never put yourself in that situation. Measure your calories and recalculate your macros so that when your weight loss plateaus, you know what to do next.

Increase Protein Intake. Increase Exercise Frequency.

Protein is good. Do not let anyone convince you otherwise. Of course, you need to maintain it within a moderate level. However, when you begin to notice your weight loss slowing down, then it is time to increase your intake of proteins. One of the best parts of the recipes mentioned in this book is that they are chock full of protein. So any time you want to have more protein, simply increase the serving sizes or portions of the food.

Moreover, make sure that you increase the amount you exercise.

Why is working out more important? Well, you are now consuming the same amount of calories that you burn. At this point, you need to burn more calories so that you can encourage weight loss.

And that is where exercises become important. You burn an incredible amount of calories through exercises. This resets the balance and you start seeing the weighing scale show progress.

Furthermore, do you remember when we talked about how you begin to lose muscles during fasting? Guess how you can reverse that and reduce the amount of muscles that you have lost?

Yep, exercise.

So make sure you have a balanced workout plan along with your fasting routine so that you can gain as many benefits as possible from your OMAD diet.

Fat Fast

There is another technique that you can use to get out of the plateau phase: a fat fast.

What exactly is a fat fast?

You know what a water fast entails. You are basically consuming mainly liquids so that you can fast for a long period of time. The long-period fasting where you fast from 24 to 72 hours is a type of water fast.

In a similar way, a fat fast is where you consume only or mainly fats. In a fat fast, you should aim to receive about 80% to 90% of your calories from fat. The remaining calories can be received from protein.

When you are engaged in a fat fast, you are recommended to have around 1,000–1,200 calories per day.

If you analyze a fat fast, then you realize that it is not actually a fast. What you are doing is ramping the amount of fats you consume and decreasing most of the other components of food. A fat fast imitates the biological properties of avoiding too much food by placing your body into a state of ketosis. When your body hits the ketosis stage, then you begin to use fats. You lower dependency on carbs.

A fat fast is specifically created to induce a calorie deficit in your body. Such a deficit is vital for your weight. A fat fast also depletes the body's reserves of carbs so that you are pushed into a state of ketosis and begin burning more fat.

If you would like to adopt a fat fast technique into your diet, then you have to ensure you boost foods that give you healthy fats and maintain such a diet for at least 3 days.

When you notice that your weight loss has gained momentum again, then you can return to your regular keto diet and continue maintaining your keto routines.

But there are a few things you must know about a fat fast.

You see, some people think that a fat fast is a quick way to enter ketosis, it could very well become an important component of their diet.

That is not a good move.

You see, fat fasting does not provide the necessary amount of protein, calories and various other micronutrients that are important for your health. This is why it is not a long-term solution for weight loss or a diet plan in and of itself. I ask you to exercise caution if you are extending a fat fast for long periods.

Apart from that one caveat, fat fasting is healthy in the short-term. It is designed for a specific purpose: accelerating your weight loss process. You should only use it for that specific purpose.

However, I have given you loads of options for recipes. So which ones should you eat to make the best use of your fat fast?

Use dishes that contain bacon, salmon, eggs, olive oil,

mayonnaise, zucchini, butter (even if it is unsalted), and nuts. There are numerous dishes you can prepare that contain the above ingredients. In many of the dishes, you can find a combination of the above ingredients. Additionally, include coffee and tea as your liquid option during your fat fast.

With that, you are ready to get back on the road to weight loss!

Conclusion

You have started your OMAD diet.

You are ready to make the most out of it.

You are now on your third or fourth day and everything is going good.

All of a sudden, you are invited to a social event. It could be someone's birthday party or a meeting between friends. You decide to attend the event. Soon, you find out that your friends or family are about to indulge in a nice juicy steak and they are hoping you join them. But that would mean you are going to have a second meal!

Gosh!

The nightmare!

Perhaps it is time to disappoint your friends or family and let them know that you won't be having that steak no matter what.

First of all, relax.

You see, this is a common problem among many people who undertake OMAD, they feel that they have to be strict about what they eat at all times.

That is not true at all.

Of course, you shouldn't indulge yourself every opportunity you get else you are defeating the purpose of an OMAD diet.

However, when it comes to social occasions, it is alright to loosen up a bit and enjoy the moment. It is not the end of the world.

When you have certain obligations, then you can go ahead and indulge yourself a bit. What you should pay attention to is the idea that you are not overindulging yourself or eating too much frequently.

You are allowed to have a second meal once in a while when the occasion calls for it. Remember that this does not mean you get to have cheat days. Rather, you might have to be part of certain social obligations. You don't want to be seen as the person who just dampened the mood of everyone at the party.

So relax and have your second meal. Just make sure that you are back on your diet the next day.

But having a second meal is just one of the concerns people have about their OMAD plan. Sometimes, it boils down to asking oneself just how many days in a week should one keep an OMAD dict. I have known people to become so obsessed with their diet that they maintain it seven days a week and then find themselves facing a serious withdrawal problem.

I am not saying that you should not keep an OMAD diet seven days a week. Rather, what you should be looking at are your goals.

What are you aiming to achieve?

If you would like to encourage a better lifestyle for yourself, then you could consider keeping an OMAD diet for 5 days a week. You will receive enough benefits during that phase to make sure that you cleanse your body, rejuvenate your cells and proteins, and find more physical and mental stability in your life.

It is true that you cannot simply indulge in high carb food during the days that you are not on your OMAD diet. You cannot have delicious and healthy salads for five days and then head over to McDonald's and pop two cheeseburgers with extra patties with a side of extra-large fries and coke on the sixth day!

You are making changes in your life and you have to maintain that change.

However, you can deviate from your OMAD diet on the sixth and seventh day. You can choose to have a nice breakfast after your 5-day OMAD plan. Perhaps even have a light lunch. And then get back to your OMAD diet again the following week.

Do note that this process has proven to be challenging for some people as they end up being reluctant to go back to their OMAD diet.

But the fact remains; you can have cheat days in your OMAD diet. The only difference is that during your cheat days, you are still eating good food. You are just having a little extra portion of it.

Remember this, you can always enjoy a delicious meal without having to resort to junk. There are plenty of food options where you might be adding a bit more carbs than usual but you are not overdosing on them.

OMAD is meant to add numerous benefits into your life. You have to enter it using a plan. When you plan out your approach, you know exactly what you would like to take from the diet.

If you are aiming to lose weight, then you know how much effort you are going to place in the OMAD process. You are not tricking yourself into thinking that things are going to be easy.

In the same way, if you are planning to maintain a healthy lifestyle then you might go a little easy on yourself. This will prevent you from thinking that OMAD is a rather scary diet to be part of.

Do note this: cheat days are going to happen.

You are going to have one of those days you cannot avoid.

My recommendation is don't avoid those days.

Enjoy yourself and live in the moment. Because you know that once you are done, you are going to get back to your diet anyway. You know that you are not straying too far from your routines and that your main goal will always be to keep a balanced and healthy diet routine.

Enjoy the process and know that you are not adopting OMAD into your life because it is just another cool fad. You are using it to better yourself.

You are creating a change that will have lasting impressions on both your physical and mental health. In fact, because one of the main components of OMAD is to maintain your stress levels, you are going to learn how to manage stress, prevent negative emotions and mental states from taking over your mind, and keep a calm demeanor. In many ways, you are becoming a master of not just your body, but your mind as well.

Progress always involves a bit of hard work. But that fact should not concern you. Rather, it should help you realize that you are an individual capable of making some incredible changes in your life.

With that, I hope you enjoy the journey you take for your OMAD diet. I sincerely hope for your success and that you find the results you seek. After all, you only get one life.

Keep it going long.

CPSIA information can be obtained
at www.ICGtesting.com
Printed in the USA
LVHW080713150719
624095LV00025B/1519/P

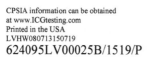